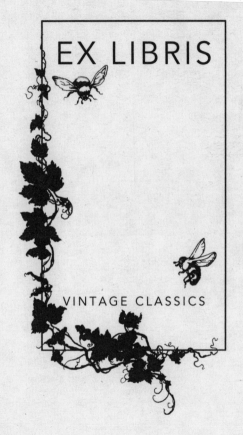

EX LIBRIS

VINTAGE CLASSICS

THE BEAUTY MYTH

Naomi Wolf was born in 1962 in San Francisco. She studied at Yale before becoming a Rhodes Scholar at New College, Oxford, and working in Edinburgh. *The Beauty Myth* was published in 1990 and became an international bestseller. Since then she has written a number of other books including *Fire with Fire, Promiscuities, Misconceptions* and her latest book, *Vagina: A New Biography*. She is also a regular contributor to the *Huffington Post* and writes cultural commentary for the *Guardian*, the *Washington Post* and *Harper's Bazaar*.

ALSO BY NAOMI WOLF

NAOMI WOLF

The Beauty Myth

How Images of Beauty are
Used Against Women

WITH AN INTRODUCTION BY
The Author

VINTAGE BOOKS
London

FOR MY PARENTS
DEOBORAH AND LEONARD WOLF

Published by Vintage 2015

5 7 9 10 8 6

The Beauty Myth was first published in Great Britain in 1990 by Chatto & Windus

This abridged edition first published in 2015 by Vintage

Vintage
Random House, 20 Vauxhall Bridge Road,
London SW1V 2SA

www.vintage-books.co.uk

Addresses for companies within The Random House Group Limited can be found at: www.randomhouse.co.uk/offices.htm

The Random House Group Limited Reg. No. 954009

A CIP catalogue record for this book is available from the British Library

ISBN 9781784870416

Printed and bound in Great Britain by
Clays Ltd, St Ives plc

Penguin Random House is committed to a sustainable future for our business, our readers and our planet. This book is made from Forest Stewardship Council® certified paper.

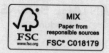

FSC

MIX
Paper from
responsible sources
FSC® C018179

CONTENTS

INTRODUCTION

When I wrote *The Beauty Myth* in 1991, I felt I was writing, to some extent, into a vacuum. Many media outlets had proclaimed that feminism – the feminism of Betty Friedan and Gloria Steinem, of NOW, was dead. Middle-class Western women, anyway, were focused on getting into the workplace, not on social revolution; the issues of working-class and poor women were far from central. News outlets repeated continually that young women rejected feminism and that 'the battles had all been won', as the cliché went.

I knew from looking at my own young peers – I was twenty-six when the book was written – that indeed the battles had not been won – but that many of them had become internalised. Though my peers no longer cared much about maintaining the perfect household – the ideal of femininity against which our mother's generation had rebelled – they were obsessed with another kind of perfection: physical perfection, as measured against fashion models and film stars. The young women around me, who should have been the brightest, most ambitious and most effective young women ever to inhabit the planet –

as they inherited the gains and analysis of feminism — were often trapped in a desperate cycle of starving themselves compulsively, or compulsively exercising, or binging and purging. Apart from the physical toll that this took, I saw the toll that these fixations took upon their ability to feel free inside their own minds — to explore themselves and their world — to fight their own battles. I saw that the epidemic of eating disorders on my own college campus as an undergraduate, and on college campuses throughout the world, and throughout the West, indeed, was a political sedative.

Since I had been fortunate enough to have studied feminist history, I realised that in every generation in which there was a great push forward by women, some ideal arose to colonise their energies and thus make sure that they did not get too far. And then, I saw, in every generation that had seen such an awakening, the next generation was told to go home — it was 'post-feminism' time — the battles had all been won. It seemed clear to me that that dynamic was what was involved with the ever-more-unattainable, ever-thinner, ever-more-surgically-enhanced quality of the images of perfection that bombarded women's sensibilities in every direction — now that women had the chance of being really free.

The initial edition of *The Beauty Myth* benefited from a lot of good fortune. It was an argument that hit at just the moment in which a generation of young women did indeed want to embrace a new version of feminism — did indeed want to analyse the unique conditions around them and take their own oppression seriously — and did indeed want to reinvigorate the discourse of feminism to take action once again, collectively as well as individually. The book was a bestseller in fourteen countries, but even more important, it was part of a new awakening of discussion and debate about many feminist topics in many new feminist voices – an awakening that writer Rebecca Walker and I, working independently, both happened to identify with a freshly coined term, The Third Wave.

Since the 1990s, feminism in the West has remained fresh, varied and vigorous; there has been a fourth wave, and I would say we are admiring the rise of a fifth. The new feminisms differ in some ways very much from the iconic feminism of the 1960s and '70s – they are more pluralistic, more tolerant, more inclusive of men, more aware of LGBTQ issues, more sophisticated about the intersection of race, class and gender, more alert to the feminist issues of the developing world. All this is a big set of advantages, and I am really proud for *The Beauty Myth*, which continues to be read, to have had a small part in this reawakening of discussion and action. But though action and awareness overall is much better for women, in some ways the 'beauty-myth' issues raised in this book have stayed the same or become worse; in other ways some have got better.

As I write today, statistics for anorexia and bulimia are exactly what they were in 1991. On some campuses 30 per cent of sorority women suffer from bulimia, making it one of the few socially transmitted mental health problems. Exercise fixations and dysmorphia – a condition in which you don't see your body in an undistorted way – are, if anything, more mainstream and widespread. The fear of ageing, among some groups of women, remains as strong as ever – new surgical technologies and lowered prices have made these interventions far more common. And eyelid-crease surgeries, nose-'refining' surgeries, dangerous skin-lightening creams, and so on – in response to globalised marketing campaigns with Western ideals – are rife in the developing world. Finally the ubiquity of pornography, which did not exist in a digitised, livestreaming format in 1991, ensures that these ideals go 'deeper' than they did in that era – as young women and young men too often feel that physical perfection is the gateway to acceptable sexuality.

On the other hand, what has become much better is the generalised awareness among women – and men – that these media ideals are both fake – indeed more fake than when I wrote this book in 1991, since then we had retouching; whereas today beauty images are simply digitally invented – and destructive. It is much more common for Girl Guides and Girl Scouts and women's magazines to discuss the artificiality and negative psychological impact of these ideas, and it is more common for women themselves to try to set up ways of reclaiming their own bodies and beauty in ways that they themselves define – from such songs as 'I am Beautiful' to such ad campaigns as the Dove campaign for Real Beauty. Editors of women's magazines, too, try to showcase more inclusive images – though the pressures on them from advertisers have remained intense. And social media – though some say it heightens pressures on young women to feel physically self-conscious – also breaks down the barrier between the consumer of media and the producer, and opens up many more models of stylishness, coolness and glamour.

On balance, I think we have come a long way. It is a great thing for young women and men today to grow up taking for granted that they are entitled to analyse and criticise the mass media ideals that are presented to them, and to define beauty, glamour and style for themselves. And it is a fantastic gift to both genders that they get to define a feminism of their own in which to do so. In that spirit, I hope you enjoy – and then make your own unique, creative and irreplaceable use of – this abridged new version of *The Beauty Myth*.

Naomi Wolf, 2015

THE BEAUTY MYTH

At last, after a long silence, women took to the streets. In the two decades of radical action that followed the rebirth of feminism in the early 1970s, Western women gained legal and reproductive rights, pursued higher education, entered the trades and the professions, and overturned ancient and revered beliefs about their social role. A generation on, do women feel free?

The affluent, educated, liberated women of the First World, who can enjoy freedoms unavailable to any women ever before, do not feel as free as they want to. And they can no longer restrict to the subconscious their sense that this lack of freedom has something to do with – with apparently frivolous issues, things that really should not matter. Many are ashamed to admit that such trivial concerns – to do with physical appearance, bodies, faces, hair, clothes – matter so much. But in spite of shame, guilt, and denial, more and more women are wondering if it isn't that they are entirely neurotic and alone but rather that something important is indeed at stake that has to do with the relationship between female liberation and female beauty.

The more legal and material hindrances women have

broken through, the more strictly and heavily and cruelly images of female beauty have come to weigh upon us. Many women sense that women's collective progress has stalled; compared with the heady momentum of earlier days, there is a dispiriting climate of confusion, division, cynicism, and above all, exhaustion. After years of much struggle and little recognition, many older women feel burned out; after years of taking its light for granted, many younger women show little interest in touching new fire to the torch.

During the past decade, women breached the power structure; meanwhile, eating disorders rose exponentially and cosmetic surgery became the fastest-growing medical specialty. During the past five years, consumer spending doubled, pornography became the main media category, ahead of legitimate films and records combined, and thirty-three thousand American women told researchers that they would rather lose ten to fifteen pounds than achieve any other goal. More women have more money and power and scope and legal recognition than we have ever had before; but in terms of how we feel about ourselves *physically,* we may actually be worse off than our unliberated grandmothers. Recent research consistently shows that inside the majority of the West's controlled, attractive, successful working women, there is a secret 'underlife' poisoning our freedom; infused with notions of beauty, it is a dark vein of self-hatred, physical obsessions, terror of aging, and dread of lost control.

It is no accident that so many potentially powerful women feel this way. We are in the midst of a violent backlash against feminism that uses images of female beauty as a political weapon against women's advancement: the beauty myth. It is the modern version of a social reflex that has been in force since the Industrial Revolution. As women released themselves from the feminine mystique of domesticity, the beauty myth took over its lost ground, expanding as it waned to carry on its work of social control.

The contemporary backlash is so violent because the ideology of beauty is the last one remaining of the old feminine ideologies that still has the power to control those women whom second wave feminism would have otherwise made relatively uncontrollable: It has grown stronger to take over the work of social coercion that myths about motherhood, domesticity, chastity, and passivity, no longer can manage. It is seeking right now to undo psychologically and covertly all the good things that feminism did for women materially and overtly.

This counterforce is operating to checkmate the inheritance of feminism on every level in the lives of Western women. Feminism gave us laws against job discrimination based on gender; immediately case law evolved in Britain and the United States that institutionalized job discrimination based on women's appearances. Patriarchal religion declined; new religious dogma, using some of the mind-altering techniques of older cults and sects, arose around age and weight to functionally supplant traditional ritual. Feminists, inspired by Friedan, broke the stranglehold on the women's popular press of advertisers for household products, who were promoting the feminine mystique; at once, the diet and skin care industries became the new cultural censors of women's intellectual space, and because of their pressure, the gaunt, youthful model supplanted the happy housewife as the arbiter of successful womanhood. The sexual revolution promoted the discovery of female sexuality; 'beauty pornography' – which for the first time in women's history artificially links a commodified 'beauty' directly and explicitly

3

to sexuality – invaded the mainstream to undermine women's new and vulnerable sense of sexual self-worth. Reproductive rights gave Western women control over our own bodies; the weight of fashion models plummeted to 23 percent below that of ordinary women, eating disorders rose exponentially, and a mass neurosis was promoted that used food and weight to strip women of that sense of control. Women insisted on politicizing health; new technologies of invasive, potentially deadly 'cosmetic' surgeries developed apace to re-exert old forms of medical control of women.

Every generation since about 1830 has had to fight its version of the beauty myth. 'It is very little to me,' said the suffragist Lucy Stone in 1855, 'to have the right to vote, to own property, etcetera, if I may not keep my body, and its uses, in my absolute right.' Eighty years later, after women had won the vote, and the first wave of the organized women's movement had subsided, Virginia Woolf wrote that it would still be decades before women could tell the truth about their bodies. In 1962, Betty Friedan quoted a young woman trapped in the Feminine Mystique: 'Lately, I look in the mirror, and I'm so afraid I'm going to look like my mother.' Eight years after that, heralding the cataclysmic second wave of feminism, Germaine Greer described 'the Stereotype': 'To her belongs all that is beautiful, even the very word beauty itself…she is a doll…I'm sick of the masquerade.' In spite of the great revolution of the second wave, we are not exempt. Now we can look out over ruined barricades: A revolution has come upon us and changed everything in its path, enough time has passed since then for babies to have grown into women, but there still remains a final right not fully claimed.

*

4

The beauty myth tells a story: The quality called 'beauty' objectively and universally exists. Women must want to embody it and men must want to possess women who embody it. This embodiment is an imperative for women and not for men, which situation is necessary and natural because it is biological, sexual, and evolutionary: Strong men battle for beautiful women, and beautiful women are more reproductively successful. Women's beauty must correlate to their fertility, and since this system is based on sexual selection, it is inevitable and changeless.

None of this is true. 'Beauty' is a currency system like the gold standard. Like any economy, it is determined by politics, and in the modern age in the West it is the last, best belief system that keeps male dominance intact. In assigning value to women in a vertical hierarchy according to a culturally imposed physical standard, it is an expression of power relations in which women must unnaturally compete for resources that men have appropriated for themselves.

'Beauty' is not universal or changeless, though the West pretends that all ideals of female beauty stem from one Platonic Ideal Woman; the Maori admire a fat vulva, and the Padung, droopy breasts. Nor is 'beauty' a function of evolution: Its ideals change at a pace far more rapid than that of the evolution of species, and Charles Darwin was himself unconvinced by his own explanation that 'beauty' resulted from a 'sexual selection' that deviated from the rule of natural selection; for women to compete with women through 'beauty' is a reversal of the way in which natural selection affects all other mammals. Anthropology has overturned the notion that females must be 'beautiful' to be selected to mate: Evelyn Reed, Elaine Morgan, and others have dismissed sociobiological assertions of innate male polygamy and female monogamy. Female higher primates are the sexual initiators; not only do they seek out and enjoy sex with many partners, but 'every nonpregnant female takes her turn at being the most desirable of all her troop. And that cycle keeps turning as long as she lives.' The inflamed pink sexual organs of primates are often cited by male sociobiologists as analogous to human arrangements relating to female 'beauty,' when in fact that is a universal, nonhierarchical female primate characteristic.

Nor has the beauty myth always been this way. Though the pairing of the older rich men with young, 'beautiful' women is taken to be somehow inevitable, in the matriarchal Goddess religions that dominated the Mediterranean from about 25,000 B.C.E. to about 700 B.C.E., the situation was reversed: 'In every culture, the Goddess has many lovers ...The clear pattern is of an older woman with a beautiful but expendable youth – Ishtar and Tammuz, Venus and Adonis, Cybele and Attis, Isis and Osiris...their only function the service of the divine "womb."' Nor is it something only women do and only men watch: Among the Nigerian Wodaabes, the women hold economic power and the tribe is obsessed with male beauty; Wodaabe men spend hours together in elaborate makeup sessions, and compete – provocatively painted and dressed, with swaying hips and seductive expressions – in beauty contests judged by women. There is no legitimate historical or biological justification for the beauty myth; what it is doing to women today is a result of nothing more exalted than the need of today's power structure, economy, and culture to mount a counteroffensive against women.

If the beauty myth is not based on evolution, sex, gender,

aesthetics, or God, on what is it based? It claims to be about intimacy and sex and life, a celebration of women. It is actually composed of emotional distance, politics, finance, and sexual repression. The beauty myth is not about women at all. It is about men's institutions and institutional power.

The qualities that a given period calls beautiful in women are merely symbols of the female behavior that that period considers desirable: *The beauty myth is always actually prescribing behavior and not appearance.* Competition between women has been made part of the myth so that women will be divided from one another. Youth and (until recently) virginity have been 'beautiful' in women since they stand for experiential and sexual ignorance. Ageing in women is 'unbeautiful' since women grow more powerful with time, and since the links between generations of women must always be newly broken: Older women fear young ones, young women fear old, and the beauty myth truncates for all the female life span. Most urgently, women's identity must be premised upon our 'beauty' so that we will remain vulnerable to outside approval, carrying the vital sensitive organ of self-esteem exposed to the air.

Though there has, of course, been a beauty myth in some form for as long as there has been patriarchy, the beauty myth in its modern form is a fairly recent invention. The myth flourishes when material constraints on women are dangerously loosened. Before the Industrial Revolution, the average woman could not have had the same feelings about 'beauty' that modern women do who experience the myth as continual comparison to a mass-disseminated physical ideal. Before the development of technologies of mass production – daguerrotypes, photographs, etc. – an ordinary woman was exposed to few such images outside the Church.

Since the family was a productive unit and women's work complemented men's, the value of women who were not aristocrats or prostitutes lay in their work skills, economic shrewdness, physical strength, and fertility. Physical attraction, obviously, played its part; but 'beauty' as we understand it was not, for ordinary women, a serious issue in the marriage marketplace. The beauty myth in its modern form gained ground after the upheavals of industrialization, as the work unit of the family was destroyed, and urbanization and the emerging factory system demanded what social engineers of the time termed the 'separate sphere' of domesticity, which supported the new labor category of the 'breadwinner' who left home for the workplace during the day. The middle class expanded, the standards of living and of literacy rose, the size of families shrank; a new class of literate, idle women developed, on whose submission to enforced domesticity the evolving system of industrial capitalism depended. Most of our assumptions about the way women have always thought about 'beauty' date from no earlier than the 1830s, when the cult of domesticity was first consolidated and the beauty index invented.

For the first time new technologies could reproduce – in fashion plates, daguerreotypes, tintypes, and rotogravures – images of how women should look. In the 1840s the first nude photographs of prostitutes were taken; advertisements using images of 'beautiful' women first appeared in mid-century. Copies of classical artworks, postcards of society beauties and royal mistresses, Currier and Ives prints, and porcelain figurines flooded the separate sphere to which middle-class women were confined.

Since the Industrial Revolution, middle-class Western women have been controlled by ideals and stereotypes as

8

much as by material constraints. This situation, unique to this group, means that analyses that trace 'cultural conspiracies' are uniquely plausible in relation to them. The rise of the beauty myth was just one of several emerging social fictions that masqueraded as natural components of the feminine sphere, the better to enclose those women inside it. Other such fictions arose contemporaneously: a version of childhood that required continual maternal supervision; a concept of female biology that required middle-class women to act out the roles of hysterics and hypochondriacs; a conviction that respectable women were sexually anesthetic; and a definition of women's work that occupied them with repetitive, time-consuming, and painstaking tasks such as needlepoint and lacemaking. All such Victorian inventions as these served a double function – that is, though they were encouraged as a means to expend female energy and intelligence in harmless ways, women often used them to express genuine creativity and passion.

But in spite of middle-class women's creativity with fashion and embroidery and child rearing, and, a century later, with the role of the suburban housewife that devolved from these social fictions, the fictions main purpose was served: During a century and a half of unprecedented feminist agitation, they effectively counteracted middle-class women's dangerous new leisure, literacy, and relative freedom from material constraints.

Though these time- and mind-consuming fictions about women's natural role adapted themselves to resurface in the postwar Feminine Mystique, when the second wave of the women's movement took apart what women's magazines had portrayed as the 'romance,' 'science,' and 'adventure' of homemaking and suburban family life, they temporarily failed. The cloying domestic fiction of 'togetherness' lost its meaning and middle-class women walked out of their front doors in masses.

So the fictions simply transformed themselves once more: Since the women's movement had successfully taken apart most other necessary fictions of femininity, all the work of social control once spread out over the whole network of these fictions had to be reassigned to the only strand left intact, which action consequently strengthened it a hundredfold. This reimposed onto liberated women's faces and bodies all the limitations, taboos, and punishments of the repressive laws, religious injunctions and reproductive enslavement that no longer carried sufficient force. Inexhaustible but ephemeral beauty work took over from inexhaustible but ephemeral housework. As the economy, law, religion, sexual mores, education, and culture were forcibly opened up to include women more fairly, a private reality colonized female consciousness. By using ideas about 'beauty,' it reconstructed an alternative female world with its own laws, economy, religion, sexuality, education, and culture, each element as repressive as any that had gone before.

Since middle-class Western women can best be weakened psychologically now that we are stronger materially, the beauty myth, as it has resurfaced in the last generation, has had to draw on more technological sophistication and reactionary fervor than ever before. The modern arsenal of the myth is a dissemination of millions of images of the current ideal; although this barrage is generally seen as a collective sexual fantasy, there is in fact little that is sexual about it. It is summoned out of political fear on the part of male-dominated institutions threatened by women's freedom, and it exploits female guilt and apprehension about our own liberation – latent fears that we might be going too far. This frantic aggregation of imagery is a collective reactionary hallucination willed into being by both men and women stunned and disoriented by the rapidity with which gender relations have been transformed: a bulwark of reassurance against the flood of change. The mass depiction of the modern woman as a 'beauty' is a contradiction: Where modern women are growing, moving, and expressing their individuality, as the myth has it, 'beauty' is by definition inert, timeless, and generic. That this hallucination is necessary and deliberate is evident in the way 'beauty' so directly contradicts women's real situation.

And the unconscious hallucination grows ever more influential and pervasive because of what is now conscious market manipulation: powerful industries – the $33-billion-a-year diet industry, the $20-billion cosmetics industry, the $300-million cosmetic surgery industry, and the $7-billion pornography industry – have arisen from the capital made out of unconscious anxieties, and are in turn able, through their influence on mass culture, to use, stimulate, and reinforce the hallucination in a rising economic spiral.

This is not a conspiracy theory; it doesn't have to be. Societies tell themselves necessary fictions in the same way that individuals and families do. Henrik Ibsen called them 'vital lies,' and psychologist Daniel Goleman describes them working the same way on the social level that they do within families: 'The collusion is maintained by directing attention away from the fearsome fact, or by repackaging its meaning in an acceptable format.' The costs of these social blind spots, he writes, are destructive communal illusions. Possibilities for women have become so open-ended that they threaten to destabilize the institutions on which a male-dominated culture has depended, and a collective panic reaction on the part of both sexes has forced a demand for counterimages.

The resulting hallucination materializes, for women, as something all too real. No longer just an idea, it becomes three-dimensional, incorporating within itself how women live and how they do not live: It becomes the Iron Maiden. The original Iron Maiden was a medieval German instrument of torture, a body-shaped casket painted with the limbs and features of a lovely, smiling young woman. The unlucky victim was slowly enclosed inside her; the lid fell shut to immobilize the victim, who died either of starvation or, less cruelly, of the metal spikes embedded in her interior. The modern hallucination in which women are trapped or trap themselves is similarly rigid, cruel, and euphemistically painted. Contemporary culture directs attention to imagery of the Iron Maiden, while censoring real women's faces and bodies.

Why does the social order feel the need to defend itself by evading the fact of real women, our faces and voices and bodies, and reducing the meaning of women to these formulaic and endlessly reproduced 'beautiful' images? Though unconscious personal anxieties can be a powerful force in the creation of a vital lie, economic necessity practically guarantees it. An economy that depends on slavery needs to promote images of slaves that 'justify' the institution of slavery. Western economies are absolutely dependent now on the continued underpayment of women. An ideology that makes women feel 'worth less' was urgently needed to counteract the way feminism had begun to make us feel worth more. This does not require a conspiracy; merely an atmosphere. The contemporary economy depends right now on the representation of women within the beauty myth. Economist John Kenneth Galbraith offers an economic explanation for 'the persistence of the view of homemaking as a "higher calling"': the concept of women as naturally trapped within the Feminine Mystique, he feels, 'has been forced on us by popular sociology, by magazines, and by fiction to disguise the fact that woman in her role of consumer has been essential to the development of our industrial society…Behavior that is essential for economic reasons is transformed into a social virtue.' As soon as a woman's primary social value could no longer be defined as the attainment of virtuous domesticity, the beauty myth redefined it as the attainment of virtuous beauty. It did so to substitute both a new consumer imperative and a new justification for economic unfairness in the workplace where the old ones had lost their hold over newly liberated women.

Another hallucination arose to accompany that of the Iron Maiden: The caricature of the Ugly Feminist was resurrected to dog the steps of the women's movement. The caricature is unoriginal; it was coined to ridicule the feminists of the nineteenth century. Lucy Stone herself, whom supporters saw as 'a prototype of womanly grace…fresh and fair as the morning,' was derided by detractors with 'the usual report' about Victorian feminists: 'a big masculine woman, wearing boots, smoking a cigar, swearing like a trooper.' As Betty Friedan put it presciently in 1960, even before the savage revamping of that old caricature: 'The unpleasant image of feminists today resembles less the feminists themselves than the image fostered by the interests who so bitterly opposed the vote for women in state after state.' Thirty years on, her conclusion is more true than ever:

That resurrected caricature, which sought to punish women for their public acts by going after their private sense of self, became the paradigm for new limits placed on aspiring women everywhere. After the success of the women's movement's second wave, the beauty myth was perfected to checkmate power at every level in individual women's lives. The modern neuroses of life in the female body spread to woman after woman at epidemic rates. The myth is undermining – slowly, imperceptibly, without our being aware of the real forces of erosion – the ground women have gained through long, hard, honorable struggle.

The beauty myth of the present is more insidious than any mystique of femininity yet: A century ago, Nora slammed the door of the doll's house; a generation ago, women turned their backs on the consumer heaven of the isolated multi-applianced home; but where women are trapped today, there is no door to slam. The contemporary ravages of the beauty backlash are destroying women physically and depleting us psychologically. If we are to free ourselves from the dead weight that has once again been made out of femaleness, it is not ballots or lobbyists or placards that women will need first; it is a new way to see.

WORK

Since men have used women's 'beauty' as a form of currency in circulation among men, ideas about 'beauty' have evolved since the Industrial Revolution side by side with ideas about money, so that the two are virtual parallels in our consumer economy. A woman looks like a million dollars, she's a first-class beauty, her face is her fortune. In the bourgeois marriage markets of the last century, women learned to understand their own beauty as part of this economy.

By the time the women's movement had made inroads into the labor market, both women and men were accustomed to having beauty evaluated as wealth. Both were prepared for the striking development that followed: As women demanded access to power, the power structure used the beauty myth materially to undermine women's advancement.

A transformer plugs into a machine at one end, and an energy source at the other, to change an unusable current into one compatible with the machine. The beauty myth was institutionalized in the past two decades as a transformer between women and public life. It links women's energy into the machine of power while altering the machine as little as possible to accommodate them; at the same time, like the transformer, it weakens women's energy at its point of origin. It does that to ensure that the machine actually scans women's input in a code that suits the power structure.

There has never been such a potentially destabilizing immigrant group asking for a fair chance to compete for access to power. Consider what threatens the power structure in the stereotypes of other newcomers. Jews are feared for their educational tradition and (for those from Western Europe) haut bourgeois memories. Asians in the United States and Great Britain, Algerians in France, and Turks in Germany are feared for their Third World patterns of grueling work at low pay. And the African-American underclass in the United States is feared for the explosive fusion of minority consciousness and rage. In women's easy familiarity with the dominant culture, in the bourgeois expectations of those who are middle class, in their Third World work habits, and in their potential to fuse the anger and loyalties of a galvanized underclass, the power structure correctly identifies a Frankenstein composite of its worst minority terrors. Beauty discrimination has become necessary, not from the perception that women will not be good enough, but that they will be, as they have been, twice as good.

And the old-boy network faces in this immigrant group a monster on a scale far greater than those it made out of other ethnic minorities, because women are not a minority. At 52.4 percent of the population, women are the majority.

Employers did not simply develop the beauty backlash because they wanted office decoration. It evolved out of fear. That fear, from the point of view of the power structure, is firmly grounded. The beauty backlash is indeed absolutely necessary for the power structure's survival.

Throughout the West, women's employment was stimulated by the widespread erosion of the industrial base and the shift to information and service technologies. Declining postwar birthrates and the resulting shortage of skilled labor means that women *are* welcome to the labor pool: as expendable, nonunionized, low-paid pink-collar-ghetto drudges. Economist Marvin Harris described women as a 'literate and docile' labor pool, and 'therefore desirable candidates for the information- and people-processing jobs thrown up by modern service industries.' The qualities that best serve employers in such a labor pool's workers are: low self-esteem, a tolerance for dull repetitive tasks, lack of ambition, high conformity, more respect for men (who manage them) than women (who work beside them), and little sense of control over their lives. At a higher level, women middle managers are acceptable as long as they are male-identified and don't force too hard up against the glass ceiling; and token women at the top, in whom the female tradition has been entirely extinguished, are useful. The beauty myth is the last, best training technique to create such a work force. It does all these things to women during work hours, and then adds a Third Shift to their leisure time.

Superwoman, unaware of its full implications, had to add serious 'beauty' labor to her *professional* agenda. Her new assignment grew ever more rigorous: the amounts of money, skill, and craft she must invest were to fall no lower than the amounts previously expected – before women breached the power structure – only from professional beauties in the display professions. Women took on all at once the roles of professional housewife, professional careerist, and professional beauty.

The Professional Beauty Qualification

Before women entered the work force in large numbers, there was a clearly defined class of those explicitly paid for their 'beauty': workers in the display professions – fashion mannequins, actresses, dancers, and higher-paid sex workers such as escorts. Until women's emancipation, professional beauties were usually anonymous, low in status, unrespectable. The stronger that women grow, the more prestige, fame, and money is accorded to the display professions: They are held higher and higher above the heads of rising women, for them to emulate.

What is happening today is that all the professions into which women are making strides are being rapidly reclassified – *so far as the women in them are concerned* – as display professions. 'Beauty' is being categorized, in professions and trades further and further afield from the original display professions, as a version of what United States sex discrimination law calls a BFOQ (a bona fide occupational qualification) and Britain calls a GOQ (a genuine occupational qualification), such as femaleness for a wet nurse or maleness for a sperm donor.

Sex equality statutes single out the BFOQ or GOQ as an *exceptional* instance in which sex discrimination in hiring is fair because the job itself demands a specific gender; as a conscious exception to the rule of equal opportunity law, it is extremely narrowly defined. What is happening now is that a parody of the BFOQ – what I'll call more specifically the PBQ, or professional beauty qualification – is being extremely *widely* institutionalized as a condition for women's hiring and promotion. By taking over in bad faith the good-faith language of the BFOQ, those who manipulate the professional beauty qualification can defend it as being nondiscriminatory with the disclaimer that it is a necessary requirement if the job is to be properly done. Since the ever-expanding PBQ has so far been applied overwhelmingly to women in the workplace and not to men, using it to hire and promote (and harass and fire) is in fact sex discrimination and should be seen as a violation of Title VII of the 1964 Civil Rights Act in the United States and the 1975 Sex Discrimination Act in Great Britain. But three new vital lies in the ideology of 'beauty' have grown during this period to camouflage the fact that the actual function of the PBQ in the workplace is to provide a risk-free, litigation-free way to discriminate against women.

Those three vital lies are: (1) 'Beauty' had to be defined as a legitimate and necessary qualification for a woman's rise in power. (2) The discriminatory purpose of vital lie number one had to be masked (especially in the United States, with its responsiveness to the rhetoric of equal access) by fitting it firmly within the American dream: 'Beauty' can be earned by any woman through hard work and enterprise. Those two vital lies worked in tandem to let the use of the PBQ by employers masquerade as a valid test of the woman's merit and extension of her professional duties. (3) The working woman was told she had to think about 'beauty' in a way that undermined, step for step, the way she had begun to think as a result of the successes of the women's movement. This last vital lie applied to individual women's lives the central rule of the myth: For every feminist action there is an equal and opposite beauty myth reaction. In the 1980s it was evident that as women became more important, beauty too became more important. The closer women come to power, the more physical self-consciousness and sacrifice are asked of them. 'Beauty' becomes the condition for a woman to take the next step. You are now too rich. Therefore, you cannot be too thin.

By the 1980s beauty had come to play in women's status-seeking the same role as money plays in that of men: a defensive proof to aggressive competitors of womanhood or manhood. Since both value systems are reductive, neither reward is ever enough, and each quickly loses any relationship to real-life values. Throughout the decade, as money's ability to buy time for comfort and leisure was abandoned in the stratospheric pursuit of wealth for wealth's sake, the competition for 'beauty' saw a parallel inflation: The material pleasures once presented as its goals – sex, love, intimacy, self-expression – were lost in a desperate struggle within a sealed economy, becoming distant and quaint memories.

The Background of the PBQ

It started in the 1960s as large numbers of educated middle-class young women began to work in cities, living alone, between graduation and marriage. A commercial sexualized mystique of the airline stewardess, the model, and the executive secretary was promoted simultaneously. The young working woman was blocked into a stereotype that used beauty to undermine both the seriousness of the work that she was doing and the implications of her new independence. Helen Gurley Brown's 1962 best seller, *Sex and the Single Girl,* was a survival map for negotiating this independence. But its title became a catchphrase in which the first term canceled out the second. The working single girl had to be seen as 'sexy' so that her work, and her singleness, would not look like what they really were: serious, dangerous, and seismic. If the working girl was sexy, her sexiness had to make her work look ridiculous, because soon the girls were going to become women.

What must this creature, the serious professional woman, look like?

Television journalism vividly proposed its answer. The avuncular male anchor was joined by a much younger female newscaster with a professional prettiness level.

That double image – the older man, lined and distinguished, seated beside a nubile, heavily made-up female junior – became the paradigm for the relationship between men and women in the workplace. Its allegorical force was and is pervasive: The qualification of professional prettiness, intended at first to sweeten the unpleasant fact of a woman assuming public authority, took on a life of its own, until professional beauties were hired to be made over into TV journalists. By the 1980s, the agents who headhunted anchors kept their test tapes under categories such as 'Male Anchors: 40 to 50,' with no corresponding category for women, and ranked women anchors' physical appearance above their delivery skills or their experience.

The message of the news team, not hard to read, is that a powerful man is an individual, whether that individuality is expressed in asymmetrical features, lines, gray hair, hairpieces, baldness, bulbousness, tubbiness, facial tics, or a wattled neck; and that his maturity is part of his power. If a single standard were applied equally to men as to women in TV journalism, most of the men would be unemployed. But the women beside them need youth and beauty to enter the same soundstage. Youth and beauty, covered in solid makeup, present the anchorwoman as generic – an 'anchorclone,' in the industry's slang. What is generic is replaceable. With youth and beauty, then, the working woman is visible, but insecure, made to feel her qualities are not unique. But, without them, she is invisible – she falls, literally, 'out of the picture.'

The situation of women in television simultaneously symbolizes and reinforces the professional beauty qualification in general: Seniority does not mean prestige but erasure – of TV anchors over forty, 97 percent, claims anchorwoman Christine Craft, are male and 'the other 3% are fortyish women who don't look their age.' Older anchorwomen go through 'a real nightmare,' she wrote, because soon they won't be 'pretty enough to do the news anymore.' Or if an anchorwoman is 'beautiful,' she is 'constantly harassed as the kind of person who had gotten her job solely because of her looks.'

The message was finalized: The most emblematic working women in the West could be visible if they were 'beautiful,' even if they were bad at their work; they could be good at their work and 'beautiful' and therefore visible, but get no credit for merit; or they could be good and 'unbeautiful' and therefore invisible, so their merit did them no good. In the last resort, they could be as good and as beautiful as you please – for too long; upon which, aging, they disappeared. This situation now extends throughout the workforce.

That double standard of appearance for men and women communicated itself every morning and every night to the nations of working women, whenever they tried to plug in to the events of 'their' world. Their window on historical developments was framed by their own dilemma. To find out what is going on in the world always involves the reminder to women that *this* is going on in the world.

In 1983, working women received a decisive ruling on how firmly the PBQ was established, and how far it could legally go. The thirty-six-year-old Craft filed suit against her ex-employers, Metromedia Inc., at Kansas City on the charge of sex discrimination. She had been dismissed on the grounds that, as Christine Craft quotes her employer, she was 'too old, too unattractive, and not deferential to men.'

Her dismissal followed months of PBQ demands made on her time and on her purse in breach of her contract, and offensive to her sense of self. She was subjected to fittings and makeovers by the hour and presented with a day-by-day chart of clothing that she would not have chosen herself and for which she was then asked to pay. None of her male colleagues had to do those things. Testimony from other anchorwomen showed that they had felt forced to quit due to Metromedia's 'fanatical obsession' with their appearance.

Other women were assigned to cover the trial. Craft was humiliated by her colleagues on camera. One suggested she was a lesbian; Diane Sawyer (who, six years later, when she won a six-figure salary, would have her appearance evaluated on *Time*'s cover with the headline IS SHE WORTH IT?) asked Craft on a national news broadcast if she really was "unique among women" in [her] lack of appearance skills.' Her employers had counted on going unchallenged because of the reaction such discrimination commonly instills in the victim of it: a shame that guarantees silence. But 'Metromedia,' she wrote defiantly, 'was wrong if they thought a woman would never admit to having been told she was ugly.'

Her account proves how this discrimination seeps in where others cannot reach, poisoning the private well from which self-esteem is drawn: 'Though I may have dismissed intellectually the statement that I was too unattractive, nonetheless in the core of my psyche I felt that something about my face was difficult, if not monstrous, to behold. It's hard to be even mildly flirtatious when you're troubled by such a crippling point of view.' An employer can't prove an employee incompetent simply by announcing that she is. But because 'beauty' lives so deep in the psyche, where sexuality mingles with self-esteem, and since it has been usefully defined as something that is continually bestowed from the outside and can always be taken away, to tell a woman she is ugly can make her feel ugly, act ugly, and, as far as her experience is concerned, *be* ugly, in the place where feeling beautiful keeps her whole.

The moral of the Christine Craft trial was that she lost: Though two juries found for her, a male judge overturned their rulings. She seems to have been blacklisted in her profession as a result of her legal fight. Has her example affected other women in her profession? 'There are thousands of Christine Crafts,' one woman reporter told me. 'We keep silent. Who can survive a blacklist?'

Defenders of Judge Stevens's ruling justified it on the grounds that it was not sex discrimination but market logic. If an anchorperson doesn't bring in the audiences, he or she has not done a good job. The nugget hidden here as it was applied to women – bring in audiences, sales, clients, or students *with her 'beauty'* – has become the legacy of the Craft case for working women everywhere.

The Law Upholds the Beauty Backlash

It could and did continue to happen to working women as the law bolstered employers with a series of Byzantine rulings that ensured that the PBQ grew ever more resilient as a tool of discrimination. The law developed a tangle of inconsistencies in which women were paralyzed: While one ruling, *Miller* v. *Bank of America,* confused sexual attraction with sexual harassment and held that the law has no part to play in employment disputes that centered on it ('attractiveness,' the court decided, being a 'natural sex phenomenon' which 'plays at least a subtle part in most personnel decisions,' and, as such, the court shouldn't delve into 'such matters'), the court in another case, *Barnes* v. *Costle,* concluded that if a woman's unique physical characteristics – red hair, say, or large breasts – were the reasons given by her employer for sexual harassment, then her personal appearance was the issue and not her gender, in which case she could not expect protection under Title VII of the 1964 Civil Rights Act. With these rulings a woman's beauty became at once her job and her fault.

Beauty provokes harassment, the law says, but it looks through men's eyes when deciding what provokes it. A woman employer may find a well-cut European herringbone twill, wantonly draped over a tautly muscled masculine flank, madly provocative, especially since it suggests male power and status, which our culture eroticizes. But the law is unlikely to see good Savile Row tailoring her way if she tells its possessor he must service her sexually or lose his job.

If, at work, women were under no more pressure to be decorative than are their well-groomed male peers in lawyer's pinstripe or banker's gabardine, the pleasure of the workplace might narrow; but so would a well-tilled field of discrimination. Since women's appearance is used to justify their sexual harassment as well as their dismissal, the statements made by women's clothing are continually, willfully misread. Since women's working clothes – high heels, stockings, makeup, jewelry, not to mention hair, breasts, legs, and hips – have already been appropriated as pornographic accessories, a judge can look at any younger woman and believe he is seeing a harassable trollop, just as he can look at any older woman and believe he is seeing a dismissable hag.

The Social Consequence of the PBQ

The professional beauty qualification works smoothly to put back into employment relations the grounds for exploitation that recent equal opportunity laws have threatened. It gives employers what they need *economically* in a female work force by affecting women *psychologically* on several levels.

The PBQ reinforces the double standard. Women have always been paid less than men for equal work, and the PBQ gives that double standard a new rationale where the old rationale is illegal.

Men's and women's bodies are compared in a way that symbolizes to both the comparison between men's and women's careers. Aren't men, too, expected to maintain a professional appearance? Certainly: They must conform to a standard that is well groomed, often uniformly clothed, and appropriate to their context. But to pretend that since men have appearance standards it means that the genders are treated equally is to ignore the fact that in hiring and promotion, men's and women's appearances are judged differently; and that the beauty myth reaches far beyond dress codes into a different realm. Male anchors, according to TV employer guidelines cited by law theorist Suzanne Levitt, are supposed to remember their 'professional image' while female anchors are cautioned to remember 'professional elegance.' The double standard for appearance is a constant reminder that men are worth more and need not try as hard.

The PBQ keeps women materially and psychologically poor. It drains money from the very women who would pose the greatest threat were they to learn the sense of entitlement bestowed by economic security: Through the PBQ, even richer women are kept away from the masculine experience of wealth. Its double standard actually makes such women poorer than their male peers, by cutting a greater swathe in the income of a female executive than in that of a male and that is part of its purpose. 'Women are punished for their looks, whereas men can go far in just a grey flannel suit,' complains, ironically, a former beauty editor of *Vogue*, who estimates that her maintenance expenses will be about $8,000 annually. Urban professional women are devoting up to a third of their income to 'beauty maintenance,' and considering it a necessary investment. Their employment contracts are even earmarking a portion of their salary for high-fashion clothing and costly beauty treatments. *New York Woman* describes a typical ambitious career woman, a thirty-two-year-old who spends 'nearly a quarter of her $60,000 income…on self-preservation.' Another 'willingly spends more than $20,000 a year' on workouts with a 'cult trainer.' The few women who are finally earning as much as men are forced, through the PBQ, to pay *themselves* significantly less than their male peers take home. It has engineered do-it-yourself income discrimination.

'Beauties' reach the peak of the possibilities open to them in early youth; so do women in the economy. The PBQ reproduces within the economy the inverted life-span of the 'beauty': Despite twenty years of the second wave of the women's movement, women's careers still are not peaking in middle and later life alongside those of men. Though business began recruiting women in the early 1970s, long enough ago to give them time for significant career advancement, only 1 to 2 percent of American upper management is female. Though half the law school graduates are women, and 30 percent of associates in private firms are female, only 5 percent of partners are women. At the top universities in the United States and Canada, the number of women full professors is also about 5 percent. The glass ceiling works to the advantage of the traditional elite, and its good working order is reinforced by the beauty myth.

One reaction to this is that older American women who have made advances within every profession are being forced to see the signs of age (the adjunct of male advancement) as a 'need' for plastic surgery. They recognize this 'need' as a professional, rather than a personal, obligation. While male peers have evidence of a generation above theirs of old, successful men who look their age, contemporary women have few such role models.

Cosmetic surgery and the ideology of self-improvement may have made women's hope for legal recourse to justice obsolete. We can better understand how insidious this development is if we try to imagine a racial discrimination suit brought in the face of a powerful technology that processes, with great pain, nonwhite people to look more white. A black employee can now charge, sympathetically, that he doesn't *want* to look more white, and should not have to look more white in order to keep his job. We have not yet begun the push toward civil rights for women that will entitle a woman to say that she'd rather look like herself than some 'beautiful' young stranger. Though the PBQ ranks women in a similar biological caste system, female identity is not yet recognized to be remotely as legitimate as racial identity (faintly though that is recognized). It is inconceivable to the dominant culture that it should respect as a political allegiance, as deep as any ethnic or racial pride, a woman's determination to show her loyalty – in the face of a beauty myth as powerful as myths about white supremacy – to her age, her shape, her self, her life.

CULTURE

Since middle-class women have been sequestered from the world, isolated from one another, and their heritage submerged with each generation, they are more dependent than men are on the cultural models on offer, and more likely to be imprinted by them. Marina Warner's *Monuments and Maidens* explains how it comes about that individual men's names and faces are enshrined in monuments, supported by identical, anonymous (and 'beautiful') stone women. That situation is true of culture in general. Given few role models in the world, women seek them on the screen and the glossy page.

This pattern, which leaves out women as individuals, extends from high culture to popular mythology: 'Men look at women. Women watch themselves being looked at. This determines not only the relations of men to women, but the relation of women to themselves.' Critic John Berger's well-known quote has been true throughout the history of Western culture, and it is more true now than ever.

Men are exposed to male *fashion* models but do not see them as *role* models. Why do women react so strongly to nothing, really – images, scraps of paper? Is their identity so weak? Why do they feel they must treat 'models' – mannequins – as if they were 'models' – paradigms? Why do women react to the 'ideal,' whatever form she takes at that moment, as if she were a non-negotiable commandment?

Heroines

It is not that women's identities are naturally weak. But 'ideal' imagery has become obsessively important to women because it was meant to become so. Women are mere 'beauties' in men's culture so that culture can be kept male. When women in culture show character, they are not desirable, as opposed to the desirable, artless ingenue. A beautiful heroine is a contradiction in terms, since heroism is about individuality, interesting and ever changing, while 'beauty' is generic, boring, and inert. While culture works out moral dilemmas, 'beauty' is amoral: If a woman is born resembling an art object, it is an accident of nature, a fickle consensus of mass perception, a peculiar coincidence – but it is not a moral act. From the 'beauties' in male culture, women learn a bitter amoral lesson – that the moral lessons of their culture exclude them.

Since the fourteenth century, male culture has silenced women by taking them beautifully apart: The catalog of features, developed by the troubadours, first paralyzed the beloved woman into beauty's silence. The poet Edmund Spenser perfected the catalog of features in his hymn the 'Epithalamion'; we inherit that catalog in forms ranging from the list-your-good-points articles in women's magazines to fantasies in mass culture that assemble the perfect women.

Culture stereotypes women to fit the myth by flatten-ing the feminine into beauty-without-intelligence or

31

intelligence-without-beauty; women are allowed a mind or a body but not both. A common allegory that teaches women this lesson is the pretty-plain pairing: of Leah and Rachel in the Old Testament and Mary and Martha in the New; Helena and Hermia in *A Midsummer Night's Dream;* Anya and Dunyasha in Chekhov's *The Cherry Orchard;* Daisy Mae and Sadie Hawkins in Dogpatch; Glinda and the Wicked Witch of the West in Oz; Veronica and Ethel in Riverdale; Ginger and Mary Ann in *Gilligan's Island;* Janet and Chrissie in *Three's Company;* Mary and Rhoda in *The Mary Tyler Moore Show;* and so forth. Male culture seems happiest to imagine two women together when they are defined as being one winner and one loser in the beauty myth.

Women's writing, on the other hand, turns the myth on its head. Female culture's greatest writers share the search for radiance, a beauty that has meaning. The battle between the overvalued beauty and the undervalued, unglamorous but animated heroine forms the spine of the women's novel. It extends from *Jane Eyre* to today's paperback romances, in which the gorgeous nasty rival has a mane of curls and a prodigious cleavage, but the heroine only her spirited eyes. The hero's capacity to see the true beauty of the heroine is his central test.

This tradition pits beautiful, vapid Jane Fairfax ('I cannot separate Miss Fairfax from her complexion') against the subtler Emma Woodhouse in Jane Austen's *Emma;* frivolous, blond Rosamond Vincy ('What is the use of being exquisite if you are not seen by the best judges?') against 'nun-like' Dorothea Casaubon in George Eliot's *Middlemarch;* manipulative, 'remarkably pretty' Isabella Crawford against self-effacing Fanny Price in Austen's *Mansfield Park;* fashionable, soulless Isabella Thorpe against Catherine Morland, unsure of herself 'where the beauty of her own sex is concerned,' in Austen's *Northanger Abbey;* narcissistic Ginevra Fanshawe ('How do I look to-night?...I know I am beautiful') against the invisible Lucy Snow ('I saw myself in the glass...I thought little of the wan spectacle') in Charlotte Bronte's *Villette;* and, in Louisa May Alcott's *Little Women,* vain Amy March, 'a graceful statue,' against tomboyish Jo, who sells her 'one beauty,' her hair, to help her family. It descends to the present in the novels of Alison Lurie, Fay Weldon, Anita Brookner. Women's writing is full to the point of heartbreak with the injustices done by beauty – its presence as well as its absence.

But when girls read the books of masculine culture, the myth subverts what those stories seem to say. Tales taught to children as parables for proper values become meaningless for girls as the myth begins its work. Take the story of Prometheus, which appears in Sullivan Reader comic-book form for third grade American children. To a child being socialized into Western culture, it teaches that a great man risks all for intellectual daring, for progress and for the public good. But as a future woman, the little girl learns that the most beautiful woman in the world was man-made, and that *her* intellectual daring brought the first sickness and death onto men. The myth makes a reading girl skeptical of the moral coherence of her culture's stories.

As she grows up, her double vision intensifies: If she reads James Joyce's *Portrait of the Artist as a Young Man,* she is not meant to question why Stephen Dedalus is the hero of his story. But in Thomas Hardy's *Tess of the D'Urbervilles* – why did the light of description fall on her, and not on any other of the healthy, untutored Wessex farm girls dancing in circles that May morning? She was seen and found beautiful, so *things happened to her* – riches, indigence, prostitution, true love, and hanging. Her life, to say the least, became interesting, while the hardhanded threshing girls around her, her friends, not blessed or cursed with her beauty, stayed in the muddy provinces to carry on the agricultural drudgery that is not the stuff of novels. Stephen is in his story because he's an exceptional subject who must and will be known. But Tess? Without her beauty, she'd have been left out of the sweep and horror of large events. A girl learns that stories happen to 'beautiful' women, whether they are interesting or not. And, interesting or not, stories do not happen to women who are not 'beautiful.'

Her early education in the myth makes her susceptible to the heroines of adult women's mass culture – the models in women's magazines. It is those models whom women usually mention first when they think about the myth.

Women's Magazines

Most commentators, like this *Private Eye* satirist, ridicule women's magazines' 'trivial' concerns and their editorial tone: 'Women's magazine triteness . . . combines knowing chatter about blowjobs with deep reservoirs of sentimentality.' Women too believe that they transmit the worst aspects of the beauty myth. Readers themselves are often ambivalent about the pleasure mixed up with anxiety that they provide. 'I buy them,' a young woman told me, 'as a form of self-abuse. They give me a weird mixture of anticipation and dread, a sort of stirred-up euphoria. Yes! Wow! I can be better starting from right this minute! Look at her! Look at *her!* But right afterward, I feel like throwing out all my clothes and everything in my refrigerator and telling my boyfriend never to call me again and blowtorching my whole life. I'm ashamed to admit that I read them every month.'

Magazines first took advertisers at the turn of the century. As suffragists were chaining themselves to the gates of the White House and of Parliament, the circulation of women's magazines doubled again. By the teens, the era of the New Woman, their style had settled into what it is today: cozy, relaxed, and intimate.

The magazines, other writers have shown, reflect shifts in women's status: Victorian magazines 'catered to a female sex virtually in domestic bondage,' but with World War I and women's participation in it, they 'quickly developed a commensurate degree of social awareness.' When the male work force came back from the trenches, the magazines returned to the home. Again in the 1940s they glamorized the world of war-production paid work and war-effort volunteer work. 'The press cooperated,' writes John Costello in *Love, Sex and War, 1939–1945,* when 'the War Manpower Commission turned to…Madison Avenue to boost its national campaign to attract first-time women workers.' Glamour, he claims, was a main tool in the enlistment campaign then, just as the beauty myth today serves government and the economy.

Though many writers have pointed out that women's magazines reflect historical change, fewer examine how part of their job is to determine historical change as well. Editors do their jobs well by reading the *Zeitgeist*; editors of women's magazines – and, increasingly, mainstream media as well – must be alert to what social roles are demanded of women to serve the interests of those who sponsor their publication. Women's magazines for over a century have been one of the most powerful agents for changing women's roles, and throughout that time – today more than ever – they have consistently glamorized whatever the economy, their advertisers, and, during wartime, the government, needed at that moment from women.

In a chapter of Betty Friedan's *The Feminine Mystique* entitled 'The Sexual Sell,' she traced how American housewives' 'lack of identity' and 'lack of purpose…[are] manipulated into dollars.' She explored a marketing service and found that, of the three categories of women, the Career Woman was 'unhealthy' from the advertisers' point of view, and 'that it would be to their advantage not to let this group get any larger…they are not the ideal type of customer. *They are too critical.*'

The marketers" reports described how to manipulate housewives into becoming insecure consumers of household products: 'A transfer of guilt must be achieved,' they said. 'Capitalize…on "guilt over hidden dirt."' Stress the 'therapeutic value' of baking, they suggested: 'With X mix in the home, you will be a different woman.' They urged giving the housewife 'a sense of achievement' to compensate her for a task that was 'endless' and 'time-consuming.' Give her, they urged manufacturers, 'specialized products for specialized tasks'; and 'make housework a matter of knowledge and skill, rather than a matter of brawn and dull, unremitting effort.' Identify your products with 'spiritual rewards,' an 'almost religious feeling,' 'an almost religious belief.' For objects with 'added psychological value,' the report concluded, 'the price itself hardly matters.' Modern advertisers are selling diet products and 'specialized' cosmetics and antiaging creams rather than household goods. In 1989, 'toiletries/cosmetics' ad revenue offered $650 million to the magazines, while 'soaps, cleansers, and polishes' yielded only one tenth that amount. So modern women's magazines now center on beauty work rather than housework: You can easily substitute in the above quotes from the 1950s all the appropriate modern counterparts from the beauty myth.

When the restless, isolated, bored, and insecure housewife fled the Feminine Mystique for the workplace, advertisers faced the loss of their primary consumer. How to make sure that busy, stimulated working women would keep consuming at the levels they had done when they had all day to do so and little else of interest to occupy them? A new ideology was necessary that would compel the same insecure consumerism; that ideology must be, unlike that of the Feminine Mystique, a briefcase-sized neurosis that the working woman could take with her to the office. To paraphrase Friedan, why is it never said that the really crucial function that women serve as aspiring beauties is *to buy more things for the body?* Somehow, somewhere, someone must have figured out that they will buy more things if they are kept in the self-hating, ever-failing, hungry, and sexually insecure state of being aspiring 'beauties.'

In the breakdown of the Feminine Mystique and the rebirth of the women's movement, the magazines and advertisers of that defunct religion were confronted with their own obsolescence. *The beauty myth, in its modern form, arose to take the place of the Feminine Mystique, to save magazines and advertisers from the economic fallout of the women's revolution.*

Imagine a women's magazine that positively featured round models, short models, old models – or no models at all, but real individual women. Let's say that it had a policy of avoiding cruelty to women, as some now have a policy of endorsing products made free of cruelty to animals. And that it left out crash diets, mantras to achieve self-hatred, and promotional articles for the profession that cuts open healthy women's bodies. And let's say that it ran articles in praise of the magnificence of visible age, displayed loving photo essays on the bodies of women of all shapes and proportions, examined with gentle curiosity the body's changes after birth and breast-feeding, offered recipes without punishment or guilt, and ran seductive portraits of men.

It would run aground, losing the bulk of its advertisers. Magazines, consciously or half-consciously, must project the attitude that looking one's age is bad because $650 million of their ad revenue comes from people who would go out of business if visible age looked good. They need, consciously or not, to promote women's hating their bodies enough to go profitably hungry, since the advertising budget for one third of the nation's food bill depends on their doing so by dieting. The advertisers who make women's mass culture possible depend on making women feel bad enough about their faces and bodies to spend more money on worthless or pain-inducing products than they would if they felt innately beautiful.

SEX

Religious guilt suppresses women's sexuality. Sex researcher Alfred Kinsey found, in the words of political analyst Debbie Taylor, that 'religious beliefs had little or no effect on a man's sexual pleasure, but could slice as powerfully as the circumcision knife into a woman's enjoyment, undermining with guilt and shame any pleasure she might otherwise experience.' Older patriarchal religions have sought, from Egyptian clitoridectomy and the Sudanese bamboo vaginal shaft and shield to the chastity belt of Germany, to control, as Rosalind Miles charges, 'all women via a technique which betrays a conscious determination to deal with the "problem" of women's sexuality by destroying it wholesale.' Beauty's new religion has taken on this tradition.

Technically, the female sexual organs *are* what the older religions feared as 'the insatiable cunt.' Capable of multiple orgasm, continual orgasm, a sharp and breathtaking clitoral orgasm, an orgasm seemingly centered in the vagina that is emotionally overwhelming, orgasm from having the breasts stroked, and of endless variations of all those responses combined, women's capacity for genital pleasure is theoretically inexhaustible.

But women's prodigious sexual capacity is not being reflected in their current sexual experience. Consistently, research figures show that the sexual revolution has left many women stranded, remote from their full ability to feel pleasure. In fact, the beauty myth hit women simultaneously with – and in backlash against – the second wave and its sexual revolution, to effect a widespread suppression of women's true sexuality. Very nearly released by the spread of contraception, legal abortion, and the demise of the sexual double standard, that sexuality was quickly restrained once again by the new social forces of beauty pornography and beauty sadomasochism, which arose to put the guilt, shame, and pain back into women's experience of sex.

Beauty pornography looks like this: The perfected woman lies prone, pressing down her pelvis. Her back arches, her mouth is open, her eyes shut, her nipples erect; there is a fine spray of moisture over her golden skin. The position is female superior; the stage of arousal, the plateau phase just preceding orgasm. On the next page, a version of her, mouth open, eyes shut, is about to tongue the pink tip of a lipstick cylinder. On the page after, another version kneels in the sand on all fours, her buttocks in the air, her face pressed into a towel, mouth open, eyes shut. The reader is looking through an ordinary women's magazine. In an ad for Reebok shoes, the woman sees a naked female torso, eyes averted. In an ad for Lily of France lingerie, she sees a naked female torso, eyes shut; for Opium perfume, a naked woman, back and buttocks bare, falls facedown from the edge of a bed; for Triton showers, a naked woman, back arched, flings her arms upward; for Jogbra sports bras, a naked female torso is cut off at the neck. In these images, where the face is visible, it is expressionless in a rictus of ecstasy. The reader understands from them that she will have to look like that if she wants to feel like that.

Beauty sadomasochism is different: In an ad for Obsession perfume, a well-muscled man drapes the naked, lifeless body of a woman over his shoulder. In an ad for Hermès perfume, a blond woman trussed in black leather is hanging upside down, screaming, her wrists looped in chains, mouth bound. In an ad for Fuji cassettes, a female robot with a playmate's body, but made of steel, floats with her genitals exposed, her ankles bolted and her face a steel mask with slits for the eyes and mouth. In an ad for Erno Laszlo skin care products, a woman sits up and begs, her wrists clasped together with a leather leash that is also tied to her dog, who is sitting up in the same posture and begging. In an American ad for Newport cigarettes, two men tackle one woman and pull another by the hair; both women are screaming. In another Newport ad, a man forces a woman's head down to get her distended mouth around a length of spurting hose gripped in his fist; her eyes are terrified. In an ad for Saab automobiles, a shot up a fashion model's thighs is captioned, 'Don't worry. It's ugly underneath.' In a fashion layout in *The Observer* (London), five men in black menace a model, whose face is in shock, with scissors and hot iron rods. In *Tatler* and *Harper's and Queen,* 'designer rape sequences (women beaten, bound and abducted, but immaculately turned out and artistically photographed)' appear. In Chris von Wangenheim's *Vogue* layout, Doberman pinschers attack a model. Geoffrey Beene's metallic sandals are displayed against a background of S and M accessories. The woman learns from these images that no matter how assertive she may be in the world, her private submission to control is what makes her desirable.

Deeper Than the Skin

In a crossover of imagery in the 1980s, the conventions of high-class pornographic photography, such as *Playboy*'s, began to be used generally to sell products to women. This made the beauty thinking that followed crucially different from all that had preceded it. Seeing a face anticipating orgasm, even if it is staged, is a powerful sell: In the absence of other sexual images, many women came to believe that they must have that face, that body, to achieve that ecstasy.

Two conventions from soft- and hard-core pornography entered women's culture: One 'just' objectifies the female body, the other does violence to it. Obscenity law is based in part on the idea that you can avoid what offends you. But the terms ordinarily used in the pornography debate cannot deal adequately with this issue. Discussions of obscenity, or nakedness, or community standards do not address the harm done to women by this development: the way in which 'beauty' joins pornographic conventions in advertising, fashion photography, cable TV, and even comic books to affect women and children. Men can choose to enter an adult bookstore; women and children cannot choose to avoid sexually violent or beauty-pornographic imagery that follows them home.

Sexual 'explicitness' is not the issue. We could use a lot more of that, if explicit meant honest and revealing; if there were a full spectrum of erotic images of uncoerced real women and real men in contexts of sexual trust, beauty pornography could theoretically hurt no one. Defenders of pornography base their position on the idea of freedom of speech, casting pornographic imagery as language. Using their own argument, something striking emerges about the representation of women's bodies: The representation is heavily censored. Because we see many versions of the naked Iron Maiden, we are asked to believe that our culture promotes the display of female sexuality. It actually shows almost none. It censors representations of women's bodies, so that only the official versions are visible. Rather than seeing images *of* female desire or that cater *to* female desire, we see mock-ups of living mannequins, made to contort and grimace, immobilized and uncomfortable under hot lights, professional set-pieces that reveal little about female sexuality. In the United States and Great Britain, which have no tradition of public nakedness, women rarely – and almost never outside a competitive context – see what other *women* look like naked; we see only identical humanoid products based loosely on women's bodies.

Beauty pornography and sadomasochism are not explicit, but dishonest. The former claims that women's 'beauty' *is* our sexuality, when the truth goes the other way around. The latter claims that women like to be forced and raped, and that sexual violence and rape are stylish, elegant, and beautiful.

The upsurge in violent sexual imagery took its energy from male anger and female guilt at women's access to power. Where beautiful women in 1950s culture got married or seduced, in modern culture the beauty gets raped. Even if we never seek out pornography, we often see rape where sex should be. Since most women repress our awareness of that in order to survive being entertained, it can take concentration to remember. According to a Screen Actors Guild study in 1989 – a year in which female leading roles made up only 14 percent of the total – a growing number of the roles for women cast them as rape victims or prostitutes. In France, TV viewers see fifteen rapes a week. That has a different effect on the audience than, for example, seeing murders: One person in four is unlikely to be murdered. But even if she avoids pornography, a woman will, by watching mainstream, middle-brow plays, films, and TV, learn the conventions of her threatened rape in detail, close up.

Rape fantasies projected into the culture are benign, we're told, even beneficial, when commentators dismiss them through what Catharine MacKinnon has satirized as 'the hydraulic model' of male sexuality (it lets off steam). Men, we are given to understand, are harmlessly interested in such fantasies; *women* are harmlessly interested in them (though many women may have rape fantasies for no more subtle psychological reason than that that image of sexuality is the primary one they witness). But what is happening now is that men and women whose private psychosexual history would not lead them to eroticize sexual violence are *learning* from such scenes to be interested in it. In other words, our culture is depicting sex as rape *so that* men and women will become interested in it.

Beauty Pornography and Sadomasochism

The current allocation of power is sustained by a flood of hostile and violent sexual images, but threatened by imagery of mutual eroticism or female desire; the elite of the power structure seem to know this consciously enough to act on it. The imposition of beauty pornography and beauty sadomasochism from the top down shows in obscenity legislation. We saw that the language of women's naked bodies and women's faces is censored. Censorship also applies to what kind of sexual imagery and information can circulate: Sexual violence against women is not obscene whereas female sexual curiosity is. British and Canadian law interprets obscenity as the presence of an erect penis, not of vulvas and breasts; and an erection, writes Susan G. Cole in *Pornography and the Sex Crisis,* is, 'according to American mores…not the kind of thing a distributor can put on the newsstands next to *Time.*' Masters and Johnson, asked in *Playboy* to comment on the average penis size, censored their findings: They 'flatly refused,' worrying that it would have 'a negative effect on *Playboy*'s readers,' and that 'everyone would walk around with a measuring stick.'

This version of censorship policed the same decades that saw the pornography industry's unparalleled growth: In Sweden, where the sale of violently misogynist pornography is defended on the grounds of freedom of expression, 'when a magazine appeared with a nude male for a centerspread, [the authorities] whisked [it] off the stalls in a matter of hours.' Women's magazine *Spare Rib* was banned in Ireland because it showed women how to examine their breasts. The Helena Rubinstein Foundation in the United States withdrew support from a Barnard women's conference because a women's magazine on campus showed 'explicit' images of women. Several art galleries banned Judy Chicago's collaborative show, *The Dinner Party,* for its depiction of the stylized genitals of heroines of women's history. The U.S. National Endowment for the Arts was attacked by Congress for sponsoring an exhibit that displayed very large penises. The Ontario Police Project P held that photos of naked women tied up, bruised, and bleeding, intended for sexual purposes, were not obscene since there were no erect penises, but a Canadian women's film was banned for a five-second shot of an erect penis being fitted with a condom. In New York subways, metropolitan policemen confiscated handmade anti-AIDS posters that showed illiterate people how to put a condom over an erect penis; they left the adjacent ads for *Penthouse,* displayed by the New York City Transit Authority, intact. Leaving aside the issue of what violent sexual imagery does, it is still apparent that there is an officially enforced double standard for men's and women's nakedness in mainstream culture that bolsters power inequities.

How Does It Work?

These images institutionalize heterosexual alienation by intervening in our fantasy lives. 'So powerful is pornography, and so smoothly does it blend in with the advertising of products…that many women find their own fantasies and self-images distorted too,' writes Debbie Taylor in *Women: A World Report.* Romantic fiction, she points out, is 'seldom sexually explicit, tending to fade out . . . when two lovers touch lips for the first time.' The same sexual evasiveness is true of nearly all dramatic presentation of mainstream culture where a love story is told. So rare is it to see sexual explicitness in the context of love and intimacy on screen that it seems our culture treats tender sexuality as if it were deviant or depraved, while embracing violent or degrading sex as right and healthy. 'This leaves,' Taylor says, 'the sexual stage,' in men's and women's minds, 'vacant, and pornographic images are free to take a starring role. The two leading actors on this stage are the sadist, played by man, and the masochist, played by woman.'

The usual discussions about pornography center on men

and what it does to their sexual attitudes toward women. But the parallel effect of beauty pornography on women is at least as important: What does that imagery do to women's sexual attitudes toward themselves? If soft-core, nonviolent, mainstream pornography has been shown to make men less likely to believe a rape victim; if its desensitizing influence lasts a long time; if sexually violent films make men progressively trivialize the severity of the violence they see against women; and if at last only violence against women is perceived by them as erotic, is it not likely that parallel imagery aimed at women does the same to women in relation to themselves? The evidence shows that it does. Wendy Stock discovered that exposure to rape imagery increased women's sexual arousal to rape and increased their rape fantasies (though it did not convince them that women liked force in sex). Carol Krafka found that her female subjects 'grew less upset with the violence [against women] the more they saw, and that they rated the material less violent' the more of it was shown to them.

The debate continues about whether classic pornography makes men violent toward women. But beauty pornography is clearly making women violent toward ourselves. The evidence surrounds us. Here, a surgeon stretches the slit skin of the breast. There, a surgeon presses with all his weight on a woman's chest to break up lumps of silicone with his bare hands. There is the walking corpse. There is the woman vomiting blood.

Sexual Battle: Profit and Glamour

Why this flood of images now? They do not arise simply as a market response to deep-seated, innate desires already in place. They arise also – and primarily – to set a sexual agenda and to *create* their versions of desire. The way to instill social values, writes historian Susan G. Cole, is to eroticize them. Images that turn women into objects or eroticize the degradation of women have arisen to counterbalance women's recent self-assertion. They are welcome and necessary because the sexes have come too close for the comfort of the powerful; they act to keep men and women apart, wherever the restraints of religion, law, and economics have grown too weak to continue their work of sustaining the sex war.

Images that flatten sex into 'beauty,' and flatten the beauty into something inhuman, or subject her to eroticized torment, are politically and socioeconomically welcome, subverting female sexual pride and ensuring that men and women are unlikely to form common cause against the social order that feeds on their mutual antagonism, their separate versions of loneliness.

Heterosexual love threatens to lead to political change: An erotic life based on nonviolent mutuality rather than domination and pain teaches firsthand its appeal beyond the bedroom. A consequence of female self-love is that the woman grows convinced of social worth.

The myth freezes the sexual revolution to bring us full circle, evading sexual love with its expensive economic price tag. The nineteenth century constrained heterosexuality in arranged marriages; today's urban overachievers sign over their sexual fate to dating services, and their libido to work: One survey found that many yuppie couples share mutual impotence. The last century kept men and women apart in rigid gender stereotypes, as they are now estranged through rigid physical stereotypes. In the Victorian marriage market, men judged and chose; in the stakes of the beauty market, men judge and choose. It is hard to love a jailer, women knew when they had no legal rights. But it is not much easier to love a judge. Beauty pornography is a warkeeping force to stabilize the institutions of a society under threat from an outbreak of heterosexual love.

Object Lessons

Glamorous rape scenes obviously eroticize the sex war. But what about nonviolent beauty pornography? The harm is apparent in the way such imagery represses female sexuality and lowers women's sexual self-esteem by casting sex as locked in a chastity belt to which 'beauty' is the only key. Since the myth began to use female sexuality to do its political work, by pairing it with 'beauty' images in a siege of repetition, it has a stronger grip on women than ever before. With sex held hostage by 'beauty,' the myth is no longer just skin deep, but goes to the core.

The myth wants to discourage women from seeing themselves unequivocally as sexually beautiful. The damage beauty pornography does to women is less immediately obvious than the harm usually attributed to pornography: A woman who knows why she hates to see another woman hanging from a meat hook, and can state her objections, is baffled if she tries to articulate her discomfort with 'soft' beauty pornography.

I once talked with other young women students about the soft-core pornography to which our college common room subscribed. I had it all wrong. I mentioned politics, symbolism, male cultural space, social exclusion, commodification. A thoughtful young woman listened intently for a while, but without a flicker of response in her eyes. 'I'll support you,' she said eventually, 'though I have no idea what you're talking about. All I know is that they make me feel incredibly bad about myself.'

The covers of soft-core magazines come close to a woman's psyche by showing versions of the models familiar to her from her own fantasy life, which is composed of images from film, TV, and women's magazines. Unlike the 'alien' whores of hard-core pornography, whose 'beauty' is less to the point than what they can be made to do, these models are a lesson to her: They are 'her' models undressed. 'Hefner's a romantic, into the beauty of it all,' says Al Goldstein, publisher of *Screw,* 'and his girls are the girls next door. My girls are the *whores* next door, with pimples and stretch marks and cheap black and white newsprint.' If those are the only two choices of sexual representation available to women, no wonder they seek beauty to the point of death.

How did this disastrous definition of sexuality arise? 'Beauty' and sexuality are both commonly misunderstood as some transcendent inevitable fact; falsely interlocking the two makes it seem doubly true that a woman must be 'beautiful' to be sexual. That of course is not true at all. The definitions of both 'beautiful' and 'sexual' constantly change to serve the social order, and the connection between the two is a recent invention. When society needed chastity from women, virginity and fidelity endowed women with beauty (religious fundamentalist Phyllis Schlafly reasserted that sex outside marriage destroyed women's beauty), and their sexuality did not exist: Peter Gay shows that Victorian women were assumed to be 'sexually anaesthetic,' and Wendy Faulkner quotes the conviction of Victorian writers that middle-class women were 'naturally frigid.' Only recently, now that society is best served by a population of women who are sexually available and sexually insecure, 'beauty' has been redefined as sex. Why? Because, unlike female sexuality, innate to all women, 'beauty' is hard work, few women are born with it, and it is not free.

The link between beauty pornography and sex is not natural. It is taken for granted that the desire to have visual access to an endless number of changing centerfolds is innately male, since that form of looking is taken to be a sublimation of men's innate promiscuity. But since men are not naturally promiscuous and women are not naturally monogamous, it follows that the truism so often asserted about beauty pornography – that men need it because they are visually aroused while women aren't – is not biologically inevitable. Men are visually aroused by women's bodies and less sensitive to their arousal by women's personalities because they are trained early into that response, while women are less visually aroused and more emotionally aroused because that is their training. This asymmetry in sexual education maintains men's power in the myth: They look at women's bodies, evaluate, move on; their own bodies are not looked at, evaluated, and taken or passed over. But there is no 'rock called gender' responsible for that; it can change so that real mutuality – an equal gaze, equal vulnerability, equal desire – brings heterosexual men and women together.

Women could probably be trained quite easily to see men first as sexual things. If girls never experienced sexual violence; if a girl's only window on male sexuality were a stream of easily available, well-lit, cheap images of boys slightly older than herself, in their late teens, smiling encouragingly and revealing cuddly erect penises the color of roses or mocha, she might well look at, masturbate to, and, as an adult, 'need' beauty pornography based on the bodies of men. And if those initiating penises were represented to the girl as pneumatically erectible, swerving neither left nor right, tasting of cinnamon or forest berries, innocent of random hairs, and ever ready; if they were presented alongside their measurements, length, and circumference to the quarter inch; if they seemed to be available to her with no troublesome personality attached; if her sweet pleasure seemed to be the only reason for them to exist – then a real young man would probably approach the young woman's bed with, to say the least, a failing heart.

But again, so what? Having been trained does not mean one cannot reject one's training. Men's dread of being objectified in the way they have objectified women is probably unfounded: If both genders were given the choice of seeing the other as a combination of sexual object and human being, both would recognize that fulfillment lies in excluding neither term. But it is the unfounded fears between the sexes that work best to the beauty myth's advantage.

Imagery that is focused exclusively on the female body was encouraged in an environment in which men could no longer control sex but had for the first time to win it. Women who were preoccupied with their own desirability were less likely to express and seek out what they themselves desired.

How to Suppress Female Sexuality

Germaine Greer wrote that women will be free when they have a positive definition of female sexuality. Such a definition might well render beauty pornography completely neutral to women. A generation later, women still lack it. Female sexuality is not only negatively defined, it is negatively constructed. Women are vulnerable to absorbing the beauty myth's intervention in our sexuality because our sexual education is set up to ensure that vulnerability. Female sexuality is turned inside out from birth, so 'beauty' can take its place, keeping women's eyes lowered to their own bodies, glancing up only to check their reflections in the eyes of men.

This outside-in eroticism is cultivated in women by three very unnatural pressures on female sexuality. The first is that little girls are not usually intimately cared for by fathers. The second is the strong cultural influence that positions women outside their bodies to look at women alone as sexual objects. The third is the prevalence of sexual violence that prohibits female sexuality from developing organically, and makes men's bodies appear dangerous.

The Sexuality of the Young: Changed Utterly?

It seems that exposure to chic violence and objectifying sexual imagery has already harmed the young. Theorists of eros have not come close to realizing the effect of beauty pornography on young people. Gloria Steinem and Susan Griffin separate pornography from eros – which makes sense if eros comes first in the psychosexual biography. Rape fantasies may be insignificant, as Barbara Ehrenreich believes, for those who grew up learning their sexuality from other human beings. But young people today did not ask for a sexuality of pleasure from distance, from danger: It was given to them. For the first time in history, children are growing up whose earliest sexual imprinting derives not from a living human being, or fantasies of their own; since the 1960s pornographic upsurge, the sexuality of children has begun to be shaped in response to cues that are no longer human. Nothing comparable has ever happened in the history of our species; it dislodges Freud. Today's children and young men and women have sexual identities that spiral around paper and celluloid phantoms: from *Playboy* to music videos to the blank female torsos in women's magazines, features obscured and eyes extinguished, they are being imprinted with a sexuality that is mass-produced, deliberately dehumanizing and inhuman.

Twelve percent of British and American parents allow their children to watch violent and pornographic films. But you don't have to watch either kind of film to tune in. Susan G. Cole notes that MTV, the rock video channel in the United States, 'appears to be conforming to pornographic standards' (the Playboy channel simply broadcasts its selections on 'Hot Rocks'). With the evolution of rock videos, both sexes sit in a room together watching the culture's official fantasy line about what they are supposed to do together – or, more often, what she is supposed to look like while he does what he does, watching her. This material, unlike the version of it in glossy magazines, moves, complicating young women's sexual anxieties in relation to beauty in a new way, as it adds levels of instruction beyond the simple pose: Now they must take notes on how to move, strip, grimace, pout, breathe, and cry out during a 'sexual' encounter. In the shift from print to videotape, their self-consciousness became three-dimensional.

Unfortunately, musical originality is not the only thing at stake: music videos set the beauty index for young women today. If the women depicted in mass culture are 'beautiful' and abused, abuse is a mark of desirability. For young men, 'beauty' is defined as that which never says no, and that which is not really human: The date-rape figures show what lessons that teaches.

In 1986, UCLA researcher Neil Malamuth reported that 30 percent of college men said they would commit rape if they could be sure of getting away with it. When the survey changed the word 'rape' into the phrase 'force a woman into having sex,' 58 percent said that they would do so. *Ms.* magazine commissioned a study funded by the National Institute for Mental Health of 6,100 undergraduates, male and female, on thirty-two college campuses across the United States. In the year prior to the *Ms.* survey, 2,971 college men had committed 187 rapes, 157 attempted rapes, 327 acts of sexual coercion, and 854 attempts at unwanted sexual contact. The *Ms.* study concluded that 'scenes in movies and TV that reflect violence and force in sexual relationships relate directly to acquaintance rape.'

Cultural representation of glamorized degradation has created a situation among the young in which boys rape and girls get raped *as a normal course of events.* The boys may even be unaware that what they are doing is wrong; violent sexual imagery may well have raised a generation of young men who can rape women without even knowing it. In 1987 a young New York woman, Jennifer Levin, was murdered in Central Park after sadomasochistic sex; a classmate remarked dryly to a friend that that was the only kind of sex that anyone he knew was having. In 1989, five New York teenagers raped and savagely battered a young woman jogger. The papers were full of stunned questions: Was it race? Was it class? No one noticed that in the fantasy subculture fed to the young, *it was normal.*

HUNGER

I saw the best minds of my generation destroyed by madness, starving...

— Allen Ginsberg, 'Howl'

There is a disease spreading. It taps on the shoulder America's firstborn sons, its best and brightest. At its touch, they turn away from food. Their bones swell out from receding flesh. Shadows invade their faces. They walk slowly, with the effort of old men. A white spittle forms on their lips. They can swallow only pellets of bread, and a little thin milk. First tens, then hundreds, then thousands, until, among the most affluent families, one young son in five is stricken. Many are hospitalized, many die.

The boys of the ghetto die young, and America has lived with that. But these boys are the golden ones to whom the reins of the world are to be lightly tossed: the captain of the Princeton football team, the head of the Berkeley debating club, the editor of the *Harvard Crimson*. Then a quarter of the Dartmouth rugby team falls ill; then a third of the initiates of Yale's secret societies. The heirs, the cream, the fresh delegates to the nation's forum selectively waste away.

The American disease spreads eastward. It strikes young men at the Sorbonne, in London's Inns of Court, in the administration of The Hague, in the Bourse, in the offices of *Die Zeit,* in the universities of Edinburgh and Tubingen and Salamanca. They grow thin and still more thin. They can hardly speak aloud. They lose their libido, and can no longer make the effort to joke or argue. When they run or swim, they look appalling: buttocks collapsed, tailbones protruding, knees knocked together, ribs splayed in a shelf that stretches their papery skin. There is no medical reason.

The disease mutates again. Across America, it becomes apparent that for every well-born living skeleton there are at least three other young men, also bright lights, who do something just as strange. Once they have swallowed their steaks and Rhine wine, they hide away, to thrust their fingers down their throats and spew out all the nourishment in them. They wander back into Maury's or '21,' shaking and pale. Eventually they arrange their lives so they can spend hours each day hunched over like that, their highly trained minds telescoped around two shameful holes: mouth, toilet; toilet, mouth.

Meanwhile, people are waiting for them to take up their places: assistantships at *The New York Times,* seats on the stock exchange, clerkships with federal judges. Speeches need to be written and briefs researched among the clangor of gavels and the whir of fax machines. What is happening to the fine young men, in their brush cuts and khaki trousers? It hurts to look at them. At the expense-account lunches, they hide their medallions of veal under lettuce leaves. Secretly they purge. They vomit after matriculation banquets and after tailgate parties at the Game. The men's room in the Oyster Bar reeks with it. One in five, on the campuses that speak their own names proudest.

How would America react to the mass self-immolation

by hunger of its favorite sons? How would Western Europe absorb the export of such a disease? One would expect an emergency response: crisis task forces convened in congressional hearing rooms, unscheduled alumni meetings, the best experts money can hire, cover stories in newsmagazines, a flurry of editorials, blame and counterblame, bulletins, warnings, symptoms, updates; an epidemic blazoned in boldface red. The sons of privilege *are* the future; the future is committing suicide.

Of course, this is actually happening right now, only with a gender difference. The institutions that shelter and promote these diseases are hibernating. The public conscience is fast asleep. Young women are dying from institutional catatonia: four hundred dollars a term from the college endowment for the women's center to teach 'self-help'; fifty to buy a noontime talk from a visiting clinician. The world is not coming to an end because the cherished child in five who 'chooses' to die slowly is a girl. And she is merely doing too well what she is expected to do very well in the best of times.

Up to one tenth of all young American women, up to one fifth of women students in the United States, are locked into one-woman hunger camps. When they fall, there are no memorial services, no intervention through awareness programs, no formal message from their schools and colleges that the society prefers its young women to eat and thrive rather than sicken and die. Flags are not lowered in recognition of the fact that in every black-robed ceremonial marches a fifth column of death's-heads.

Some women's magazines report that 60 percent of American women have serious trouble eating. The majority of middle-class women in the United States, it appears, suffer a version of anorexia or bulimia; but if anorexia is defined as a compulsive fear of and fixation upon food, perhaps most Western women can be called, twenty years into the backlash, mental anorexics.

What happened? Why now? The first obvious clue is the progressive chiseling away of the Iron Maiden's body over this century of female emancipation, in reaction to it. Until seventy-five years ago in the male artistic tradition of the West, women's natural amplitude was their beauty; representations of the female nude reveled in women's lush fertility. Various distributions of sexual fat were emphasized according to fashion – big, ripe bellies from the fifteenth to the seventeenth centuries, plump faces and shoulders in the early nineteenth, progressively generous dimpled buttocks and thighs until the twentieth – but never, until women's emancipation entered law, this absolute negation of the female state that fashion historian Ann Hollander in *Seeing Through Clothes* characterizes, from the point of view of any age but our own, as 'the look of sickness, the look of poverty, and the look of nervous exhaustion.'

Dieting and thinness began to be female preoccupations when Western women received the vote around 1920; between 1918 and 1925, 'the rapidity with which the new, linear form replaced the more curvaceous one is startling.' In the regressive 1950s, women's natural fullness could be briefly enjoyed once more because their minds were occupied in domestic seclusion. But when women came en masse into male spheres, that pleasure had to be overridden by an urgent social expedient that would make women's bodies into the prisons that their homes no longer were.

The great weight shift must be understood as one of the major historical developments of the century, a direct solution to the dangers posed by the women's movement and economic and reproductive freedom. Dieting is the most potent political sedative in women's history; a quietly mad population is a tractable one. Researchers S. C. Wooley and O. W. Wooley confirmed what most women know too well – that concern with weight leads to 'a virtual collapse of self-esteem and sense of effectiveness.' Researchers J. Polivy and C. P. Herman found that 'prolonged and periodic caloric restriction' resulted in a distinctive personality whose traits are 'passivity, anxiety and emotionality.'

It is those traits, and not thinness for its own sake, that the dominant culture wants to create in the private sense of self of recently liberated women in order to cancel out the dangers of their liberation.

Just as the thin Iron Maiden is not actually beautiful, anorexia, bulimia, even compulsive eating, symbolically understood, are not actually diseases. They *begin,* as Susie Orbach notes, as sane and mentally healthy responses to an insane social reality: that most women can feel good about themselves only in a state of permanent semistarvation. The anorexic refuses to let the official cycle master her: By starving, she masters it. A bulimic may recognize the madness of the hunger cult, its built-in defeat, its denial of pleasure. A mentally healthy person will resist having to choose between food and sexuality – sexuality being bought, today, by maintenance of the official body. By vomiting, she gets around the masochistic choice. Eating diseases are often interpreted as symptomatic of a neurotic need for control. But surely it is a sign of mental health to try to control something that is trying to control you, especially if you are a lone young woman and it is a massive industry fueled by the needs of an entire determined world order.

Self-defense is the right plea when it comes to eating disasters; not insanity. Self-defense bears no stigma, whereas madness is a shame.

Victorian female hysteria, mysterious at the time, makes sense now that we see it in the light of the social pressures of sexual self-denial and incarceration in the home. Anorexia should be as simple to understand. What hysteria was to the nineteenth-century fetish of the asexual woman locked in the home, anorexia is to the late-twentieth-century fetish of the hungry woman.

Sex, food, and flesh; it is only political ideology – not health, not men's desires, not any law of loveliness – that keeps women from believing we can have all three. Young women believe what they have no memory to question, that they may not have sex, food, and flesh in any abundance; that those three terms cancel each other out.

The Third Wave: Frozen in Motion

If we look at most young women's inert relationship to feminism, we can see that with anorexia and bulimia, the beauty myth is winning its offensive. Where are the women activists of the new generation, the fresh blood to infuse energy into second-wave burnout and exhaustion? Why are so many so quiet? On campuses, up to a fifth of them are so quiet because they are starving to death. Starving people are notorious for a lack of organizational enthusiasm. Roughly another 50 percent are overcome with a time-devouring and shameful addiction to puking their guts out in the latrines of the major centers of higher learning. The same young women who would seem to be its heiresses are not taking up the banner of the women's movement for perhaps no more profound reason than that many of them are too physically ill to do much more than cope with immediate personal demands. And on a mental level, the epidemic of eating disorders may affect women of this generation in such a way as to make feminism seem viscerally unconvincing: Being a woman is evidently nothing to be up in arms about; it makes you hungry, weak, and sick.

Young girls and women are seriously weakened by inheriting the general fallout of two decades of the beauty myth's backlash. But other factors compound these pressures on young women so intensely that the surprise is not how many do have eating diseases, but that any at all do not.

The pressure of beauty pornography and the pressures of achievement combine to strike young women where they are most vulnerable: in their exploration of their sexuality in relation to their sense of their own worth. Beauty pornography makes an eating disease seem inevitable, even desirable, if a young woman is to consider herself sexual and valuable: Robin Lakoff and Raquel Scherr in *Face Value* found in 1984 that 'among college women, "modern" definitions of beauty – health, energy, self-confidence' – prevailed. 'The bad news' is that they all had 'only one overriding concern: the shape and weight of their bodies. They all wanted to lose 5–25 pounds, even though most [were] not remotely overweight. They went into great detail about every flaw in their anatomies, and told of the great disgust they felt every time they looked in the mirror.' The 'great disgust' they feel comes from learning the rigid conventions of beauty pornography before they learn their own sexual value; in such an atmosphere, eating diseases make perfect sense.

The Anorexic/Pornographic Generation

When women of different ages do have the rare opportunity to talk, the gap between older women and those of the anorexic/pornographic generations causes grave mistranslations. 'This is what I say to get their attention,' says Betty Friedan of her college audiences.

> 'How many of you have ever worn a girdle?' And they laugh. Then I say…'It used to be that being a woman in the United States meant that you encased your flesh in rigid plastic casing that made it difficult to breathe and difficult to move, but you weren't supposed to notice that. You didn't ask why you wore the girdle, and you weren't supposed to notice red welts on your belly when you took it off at night.' And then I say, 'How can I expect you to know what it felt like when you have never worn anything under your blue jeans except panty hose, or little bikinis?' That gets to them. Then I explain how far we've come, where we are now, and why they have to start saying, 'I am a feminist.'

For many young women in Friedan's audience, the girdle is made of their own flesh. They can't take it off at night. The 'little bikinis' have not brought this generation heedless bodily freedom; they have become props that superimpose upon the young women chic pseudosexual scenarios that place new limits on what they can think, how they can move, and what they can eat. The backlash does to young women's minds, so much more free, potentially, than any ever before, what corsets and girdles and gates on universities no longer can. The post-1960 daughter sees more images of impossibly 'beautiful' women engaged in 'sexual' posturing in one day than her mother saw throughout adolescence: She needs to be shown more if she is to know her place. By saturation in imagery, the potential explosiveness of this generation is safely defused.

VIOLENCE

One must suffer to be beautiful.

– French Proverb

Women must labour to be beautiful.

– W. B. Yeats

Unto the woman He said, I will greatly multiply thy pain and thy travail; in pain thou shalt bring forth children; and thy desire shall be to thy husband, and he shall rule over thee.

– Genesis 3:16

Hunger makes women's bodies hurt them, and makes women hurt their bodies. Studies of abusers show that violence, once begun, escalates. Cosmetic surgery is the fastest-growing 'medical' specialty. More than two million Americans, at least 87 percent of them female, had undergone it by 1988, a figure that had tripled in two years. Throughout the 1980s, as women gained power, unprecedented numbers of them sought out and submitted to the knife. Why surgery? Why now?

From the beginning of their history until just before the 1960s, women's gender caused them pain. Because of puerperal fever and childbed complications, giving birth was cruelly painful until the invention of chloroform in 1860, and mortally dangerous until the advent of antisepsis in the 1880s. Afterward, sex still carried the risk of an illegal abortion, with its dangers of hemorrhage, perforated uterus, and death by blood poisoning. 'Labor' for women has meant childbirth, so that work, sex, love, pain, and death, over the centuries, intertwined into a living knot at the center of female consciousness: Love hurt, sex could kill, a woman's painful labor was a labor of love. What would be masochism in a man has meant survival for a woman.

Sex began to lose its sting in 1965, when in the case of *Griswold* v. *Connecticut* the U.S. Supreme Court legalized the sale of contraceptives and the Pill was widely prescribed. It hurt even less from the late 1960s until the late 1980s, when safe abortion was legalized in most Western countries. As women entered the paid work force and lost their dependence on sexual barter for survival, it hurt less still. Changing social mores and the women's movement's championing of female sexuality began to make it imaginable that the pleasure their sex gave women might finally and forever outweigh the pain. The strands of sex and pain in women at last began to separate.

In the strange new absence of female pain, the myth put beauty in its place. For as far back as women could remember, something had hurt about being female. As of a generation ago, that became less and less true. But neither women nor the masculine social order could adapt so abruptly to a present in which femaleness was not characterized and defined by pain. Today, what hurts is beauty.

Cosmetic surgery processes the bodies of woman-made women, who make up the vast majority of its patient pool, into man-made women. It took over the regions of the female mind left unpoliced when female sexuality stopped hurting, and exploited our willingness to heed an authoritarian voice that announces – as we uneasily try out the alien state of the pain-free women – Not so fast.

The Walking Wounded

The cosmetic surgery industry is expanding by manipulating ideas of health and sickness. There is a clear historical precedent for what the surgeons are doing. 'Healthy' and 'diseased,' as Susan Sontag points out in *Illness as Metaphor,* are often subjective judgments that society makes for its own purposes. Women have long been defined as sick as a means of subjecting them to social control. What the modern Surgical Age is doing to women is an overt reenactment of what nineteenth-century medicine did to make well women sick and active women passive. The surgical industry has taken over for its own profit motives the ancient medical attitude, which harks back to classical Greece but reached its high point in the Victorian female cult of invalidism, which defines normal, healthy female physiology, drives, and desires as pathological. 'In the traditions of Western thought,' write Deirdre English and Barbara Ehrenreich in *Complaints and Disorders: The Sexual Politics of Sickness,* 'man represents wholeness, strength and health. Woman is a "misbegotten man," weak and incomplete.' Historian Jules Michelet refers to women as 'the walking wounded.'

The Surgical Age took over from the institutionalization of female 'mental illness,' which had in turn overtaken the institutionalization of nineteenth-century hysteria, each phase of medical coercion consistently finding new ways to determine that what is female is sick. As English and Ehrenreich put it: 'Medicine's prime contribution to sexist ideology has been to describe women as sick, and as potentially sickening to men.' The 'vital lie' that equates femaleness with disease has benefited doctors in each of these three phases of medical history, guaranteeing them 'sick' and profitable patients wherever middle-class women can be found. The old edifice of medical coercion of women, temporarily weakened when women entered medical schools in significant numbers, has gained reinforcements from the beauty doctors of the Surgical Age.

Health

The nineteenth-century version of medical coercion looks quaint to us: How could women have been made to believe that menstruation, masturbation, pregnancy, and menopause were diseases? But as modern women are being asked to believe that parts of our normal, healthy bodies are diseased, we have entered a new phase of medical coercion that is so horrific that no one wants to look at it at all.

The purpose of the Victorian cult of female invalidism was social control. It too was a double symbol, like 'beauty': Subjectively, women invalids exerted through it the little power they had, escaped onerous sexual demands and dangerous childbirth, and received attention from responsive doctors. But for the establishment, it was a political solution as useful as the Iron Maiden. As French writer Catherine Clement puts it: 'Hysteria [was] tolerated because in fact it has no power to effect cultural change; it is much safer for the patriarchal order to encourage and allow discontented women to express their wrongs through psychosomatic illness than to have them agitating for economic and legal rights.' Social pressure demanded that leisured, educated, middle-class women preempt trouble by being sick, and the enforced hypochondria felt to the sufferer like real illness. For similar reasons today, social pressure requires that women preempt the implications of our recent claim to our bodies by feeling ugly, and that forcibly lowered self-esteem looks to the sufferer like real 'ugliness.'

A century ago, normal female activity, especially the kind that would lead women into power, was classified as ugly and sick. If a woman read too much, her uterus would 'atrophy.' If she kept on reading, her reproductive system would collapse and, according to the medical commentary of the day, 'we should have before us a repulsive and useless hybrid.' Menopause was depicted as a terminal blow, 'the death of the woman in the woman': 'The end of a woman's reproductive life was as profound a mental upheaval as the beginning,' producing, like the modern waning of 'beauty,' 'a distinct shock to the brain.' Then as now, though with a different rationalization, menopause was represented as causing the feeling that 'the world…is turned upside down, that everything is changed, or that some very dreadful but undefined calamity has happened or is about to happen.'

Participation in modernity, education, and employment was portrayed as making Victorian women ill: 'warm apartments, coal-fires, gas-lights, late hours, rich food,' turned them into invalids, as today, as the skin cream copy puts it, 'central heating, air pollution, fluorescent lights, etc.' make us 'ugly.' Victorians protested women's higher education by fervidly imagining the damage it would do to their reproductive organs; Friedrich Engels claimed that 'protracted work frequently causes deformities of the pelvis,' and it was taken for granted that 'the education of women would sterilize them' and make them sexually unattractive: 'When a woman displays scientific interest, then there is something out of order in her sexuality.' The Victorians insisted that freedom from the 'separate sphere' impaired womanhood, just as we are asked to believe that freedom from the beauty myth impairs beauty.

In 1985, Eugenia Chandris in *The Venus Syndrome* called big hips and thighs 'a medical problem'; looking at the Paleolithic fertility figures, she committed the solecism of saying that 'the problem has troubled women ever since.' 'The problem,' of course, has only troubled women since it has been called a problem – that is, within living memory. Female fat is characterized as if it were not only dead, but carcinogenic: 'proliferating cells,' breeding more death. The Victorians defined all reproductive activity as illness; today's beauty surgeons define as illness all evidence on the body of its reproductive activity – stretch marks, sagging breasts, breasts that have nursed, and the postpartum weight that accumulates, in every culture, at about ten pounds per pregnancy. Education, of course, never affected a woman's ovaries, just as maternal breasts lose no feeling; nursing *is* erotic.

Is 'Health' Healthful?

How healthy is the Surgical Age? Smoking is on the decline in all groups but young women; 39 percent of all women who smoke say they smoke to maintain their weight; one quarter of those will die of disease caused by cigarette smoking – though, to be fair, the dead women's corpses will weigh on average four pounds less than will the bodies of the living nonsmokers. Capri cigarettes are advertised as 'the slimmest slim.' The late Rose Cipollone, whose husband sued the tobacco industry for her death from lung cancer, started smoking as a teenager because 'I thought I was going to be glamorous or beautiful.'

Liquid fasts have caused at least sixty deaths in the United States, and their side effects include nausea, hair loss, dizziness, and depression. Compulsive exercise causes sports anemia and stunted growth. Breast implants make cancer detection more difficult. Women delay mammograms for fear of losing a breast and becoming 'only half a woman.'

The prime of life, the decades from forty to sixty – when many men but certainly most women are at the height of their powers – are cast as men's peak and women's decline (an especially sharp irony since those years represent women's sexual peak and men's sexual decline). This double standard is not based on health differences between middle-aged men and women, but on the artificial inequality of the beauty myth. The hypocrisy of the use of 'health' as a gloss for the Surgical Age is that the myth's true message is that a woman should live hungry, die young, and leave a pretty corpse.

The Surgical Age's definition of female 'health' is not healthy. Are those aspects defined as 'diseased' actually sick?

You could see the signs of female aging as diseased, especially if you had a vested interest in making women too see them your way. Or you could see that if a woman is healthy she lives to grow old; as she thrives, she reacts and speaks and shows emotion, and grows into her face. Lines trace her thought and radiate from the corners of her eyes after decades of laughter, closing together like fans as she smiles. You could call the lines a network of 'serious lesions,' or you could see that in a precise calligraphy, thought has etched marks of concentration between her brows, and drawn across her forehead the horizontal creases of surprise, delight, compassion, and good talk. A lifetime of kissing, of speaking and weeping, shows expressively around a mouth scored like a leaf in motion. The skin loosens on her face and throat, giving her features a setting of sensual dignity; her features grow stronger as she does. She has looked around in her life, and it shows. When gray and white reflect in her hair, you could call it a dirty secret or you could call it silver or moonlight. Her body fills into itself, taking on gravity like a bather breasting water, growing generous with the rest of her. The darkening under her eyes, the weight of her lids, their minute crosshatching, reveal that what she has been part of has left in her its complexity and richness. She is darker, stronger, looser, tougher, sexier. The maturing of a woman who has continued to grow is a beautiful thing to behold.

Or, if your ad revenue or your seven-figure salary or your privileged sexual status depend on it, it is an operable condition.

Whatever is deeply, essentially female – the life in a woman's expression, the feel of her flesh, the shape of her breasts, the transformations after childbirth of her skin – is being reclassified as ugly, and ugliness as disease. These qualities are about an intensification of female power, which explains why they are being recast as a diminution of power. At least a third of a woman's life is marked with aging; about a third of her body is made of fat. Both symbols are being transformed into operable conditions – *so that* women will only feel healthy if we are two thirds of the women we could be. How can an 'ideal' be about women if it is defined as how much of a female sexual characterisic *does not* exist on the woman's body, and how much of a female life *does not* show on her face?

Profit

It cannot be about women, for the 'ideal' is not about women but about money. The current Surgical Age is, like the Victorian medical system, impelled by easy profits. The cosmetic surgery industry in the United States grosses $300 million every year, and is growing annually by 10 percent. But as women get used to comfort and freedom, it cannot continue to count on profit from women's willingness to suffer for their sex. A mechanism of intimidation must be set in place to maintain that rate of growth, higher than that of any other 'medical specialty.' Women's pain threshold has to be raised, and a new sense of vulnerability imbedded in us, if the industry is to reap the full profit of their new technology acting on old guilt. The surgeons' market is imaginary, since there is nothing wrong with women's faces or bodies that social change won't cure; so the surgeons depend for their income on warping female self-perception and multiplying female self-hatred.

If women suddenly stopped feeling ugly, the fastest-growing medical specialty would be the fastest dying. In many states of the United States, where cosmetic surgeons (as opposed to plastic surgeons, who specialize in burns, trauma, and birth defects) can be any nonspecialist M.D., it would be back to mumps and hemorrhoids for the doctors, conditions that advertising cannot exacerbate. They depend for their considerable livelihood on selling women a feeling of terminal ugliness. If you tell someone she has cancer, you cannot create in her the disease and its agony. But tell a woman persuasively enough that she is ugly, you do create the 'disease,' and its agony is real. If you wrap up your advertisement, alongside an article promoting surgery, in a context that makes women feel ugly, and leads us to believe that other women are competing in this way, then you have paid for promoting a disease that you alone can cure.

Safeguards

Medical coercion in service of a vital lie is less regulated than legitimate medicine. In the nineteenth century, sexual surgery was risky and unscientific, with few legal checks. Patients were more likely, until around 1912, to be harmed by medical intervention than helped. Little, according to today's standards, was known about how the body worked, and strange experiments on women's reproductive organs were common. The American Medical Association had no legal control over who could call himself a doctor. Doctors had virtually free rein to peddle opiate-based, addictive snake oils, and miracle cures for vague female maladies.

The new atrocities are flourishing without intervention from the institutions that promise to safeguard the welfare of citizens. In a sexual double standard as to who receives consumer protection, it seems that if what you do is done to women in the name of beauty, you may do what you like. It is illegal to claim that something grows hair, or makes you taller, or restores virility, if it does not. It is difficult to imagine that the baldness remedy Minoxidil would be on the market if it had killed nine French and at least eleven American men. In contrast, the longterm effects of Retin-A are still unknown – Dr Stuart Yuspa of the National Cancer Institute refers to its prescription as 'a human experiment' – and the Food and Drug Administration has not approved it; yet dermatologists are prescribing it to women at a revenue of over $150 million a year.

In Great Britain, objective-sounding organizations have sprung up which specialize in cosmetic surgery – and make use on their literature of the winged staff and serpents of Asclepius, god of healing and of the medical profession, giving women the impression that they will get impartial information, when what they do is lobby over the phone, through medically untrained 'counselors,' for new patients. In the United States, it was not until 1989, ten years into the Surgical Age, that a congressional hearing was convened by Congressman Ron Wyden (Democrat, Oregon), to investigate what one witness called 'the last refuge of freebooters charging what the market will bear' and their advertising, which is 'often misleading and false...preying on the insecurities of American women.' Testimony accused the Federal Trade Commission of a failure to regulate the 'profession,' and blamed it for permitting advertising in the 1970s and then abandoning responsibility for what the ads had wrought. An M.D/D.P.S. is 'board-certified' by the American Board of Plastic Surgery, and therefore trained; but an American woman who is told that it is her burden to ensure that the surgeon is 'board-certified' is unlikely to know that there are over one hundred different 'boards' with official-sounding names that go unregulated. Fully 90 percent of cosmetic surgery in the United States is performed in unregulated doctors'' offices. Finally, asserted the congressional testimony, 'there is no standard method for preoperative screening,' so any woman is operable. What did Congress do about the situation once it was staring them in the face? Nothing: The legislation proposed after Congress saw 1,790 pages of shocking testimony is, says Dr Steve Scott, spokesman for Congressman Wyden's office, more than a year afterward, 'on hold.' Why? Because it happens to women for beauty, so it is not serious.

Sexual Surgery

It is not coincidental that breast surgery is expanding at a time when female sexuality is such a threat. That was true in Victorian times as well, when doctors treated amenorrhea by placing leeches directly on the vagina or cervix, and cauterized the uterus for discharge with chromic acid. 'The operation…is not what's important,' says a rhinoplasty patient, as Victorian women's 'mental agony and physical torture was accounted nothing.' Surgeons are becoming media stars. 'Glamour and prestige' came to surround the gynecological surgeon, and doctors often advised surgery where less dramatic measures were enough. Ovariotomy 'became a fashionable operation in spite of a mortality rate sometimes as high as 40%. *Not only the diseased ovary but the healthy, normal ovary fell prey to the sexual surgeons*' (italics added). One has only to open a cosmetic surgery brochure to see how very normal and healthy are the breasts now 'prey to the sexual surgeons.'

The artificial reconstruction of the breast may now have become eroticized for women too. It is only after two decades of beauty pornography curtailing female sexuality that a sexually dead breast can be seen and felt to be 'better' than one that is sexually alive. The same tacit censorship that edits images of women's faces and body shapes also edits images of the female breast, keeping women ignorant about what breasts are actually like. Culture screens breasts with impeccable thoroughness, almost never representing those that are soft, or asymmetrical, or mature, or that have gone through the changes of pregnancy. Looking at breasts in culture, one would have little idea that real breasts come in as many shapes and variations as there are women. Since most women rarely if ever see or touch other women's breasts, they have no idea what they feel like, or of the way they move and shift with the body, or of how they really look during lovemaking. Women of all ages have a fixation – sad in the light of how varied women's breasts really are in texture – on 'pertness' and 'firmness.' Many young women suffer agonies of shame from their conviction that they alone have stretch marks. Since beauty censorship keeps women in profound darkness about other women's real bodies, it is able to make virtually any woman feel that her breasts alone are too soft or low or sagging or small or big or weird or wrong, and to steal from her the full and exquisite eroticism of the nipple.

Freud believed that repression of the libido made civilization; civilization depends at the moment on the repression of female libido: In 1973, *Psychology Today* reports, one fourth of American women surveyed were unhappy with the size or shape of their breasts. By 1986, the number had risen to a third; it was not women's breasts that had changed in the meantime.

Choice

'Beauty's' pain is trivial since it is assumed that women freely choose it. That conviction is what keeps people from seeing that what the Surgical Age is doing to women is human rights abuse. The hunger, the nausea, and surgical invasions of the beauty backlash are political weapons. Through them, a widespread political torture is taking place among us.

When a class of people is denied food, or forced to vomit regularly, or repeatedly cut open and stitched together to no medical purpose, we call it torture. Are women less hungry, less bloody, if we act as our own torturers?

Most people will say yes, since women do it to themselves, and it is something that must be done. But it is illogical to conclude that there is a different quality to blood or hunger or second-degree burning because it was 'chosen.' Nerve endings cannot tell who has paid for the slicing; a raw dermis is not comforted by the motive behind its burning. People respond illogically when confronted with beauty's pain since they believe that masochists deserve the pain they get because they enjoy it.

Women's desperation for beauty is derided as narcissism; but women are desperate to hold on to a sexual center that no one threatens to take away from men, who keep sexual identity in spite of physical imperfections and age. Men do not hear in the same way the message that time is running out, and that they will never again be stroked and admired and gratified. Let a man imagine himself living under that threat before he calls women narcissistic. Fighting for 'beauty,' many of us understandably believe we are fighting for our lives, for life warmed by sexual love.

With the threat of lost love comes the threat of invisibility. Extreme age shows the essence of the myth's inequality: The world is run by old men; but old women are erased from the culture. A banned or ostracized person becomes a nonperson. Ostracism and banning are effective, and leave no proof of coercion: no bars, no laws, no guns. South African activist Beyers Naude said on British television that 'a banning order can easily lead to people breaking down.' Few can bear being treated as if they are invisible. Women have face-lifts in a society in which women without them appear to vanish from sight.

Surgical Futures

The Victorians' definition of operable kept expanding. 'Moral insanity,' like ugliness, was a 'definition that could be altered to take in almost any kind of behavior regarded as abnormal or disruptive by community standards,' writes Elaine Showalter. 'Asylums opened for "young women of ungovernable temper...sullen, wayward, malicious, defying all domestic control; or who want that restraint over their passions without which the female character is lost."' So does our definition of operable keep expanding, for the same reasons. In the 1970s, intestinal bypass surgery (in which the intestines are sealed off for weight loss) was invented and it multiplied until, by 1983, there were fifty thousand such operations performed a year. Jaw clamps (in which the jaw is wired together for weight loss) were also introduced in the feminist 1970s, and stomach stapling (in which the stomach is sutured together for weight loss) began in 1976. 'As time went on,' reports *Radiance,* 'the criteria for acceptance became looser and looser until now anyone who is even moderately plump can find a cooperative surgeon.' Women of 154 pounds have had their intestines stapled together. Though the doctor who developed it restricted the procedure to patients more than 100 pounds overweight, the FDA approved it for 'virtually anyone who wants it.'

Liposuction shows the way to the future: It is the first of many procedures to come for which all women will be eligible by virtue of being women.

The Iron Maiden Breaks Free

Women are in jeopardy from our current misunderstanding of the Iron Maiden. We still believe that there is some point where surgery is constrained by a natural limit, the outline of the 'perfect' human female. That is no longer true. The 'ideal' has never been about the bodies of women, and from now on technology can allow the 'ideal' to do what it has always sought to do: leave the female body behind altogether to clone its mutations in space. The human female is no longer the point of reference.

The 'ideal' has become at last fully inhuman. One model points out in *Cosmopolitan* that 'the ideal today is a muscular body with big breasts. Nature doesn't make women like that.' And, in fact, women no longer see versions of the Iron Maiden that represent the natural female body. 'Today,' says Dr Stephen Herman of Albert Einstein College of Medicine Hospital, 'I think, almost every popular model has had some type of breast augmentation operation.' 'Many models,' another women's magazine concedes, 'now regard a session with the plastic surgeon as part of their job requirement.' Fifty million Americans watch the Miss America pageant; in 1989 five contestants, including Miss Florida, Miss Alaska, and Miss Oregon, were surgically reconstructed by a single Arkansas plastic surgeon. Women are comparing themselves and young men are comparing young women with a new breed that is hybrid nonwoman. Women's natural attractions were never the aim of the beauty myth, and technology has finally cut the cord. She says, I feel bad about this; he cuts. She says, What about this here; he cuts.

Whatever the future threatens, we can be fairly sure of this: Women in our 'raw' or 'natural' state will continue to be shifted from category 'woman' to category 'ugly,' and shamed into an assembly-line physical identity. As each woman responds to the pressure, it will grow so intense that it will become obligatory, until no self-respecting woman will venture outdoors with a surgically unaltered face. The free market will compete to cut up women's bodies more cheaply, if more sloppily, with no-frills surgery in bargain basement clinics. In that atmosphere, it is a matter of time before they reposition the clitoris, sew up the vagina for a snugger fit, loosen the throat muscles, and sever the gag reflex. Los Angeles surgeons have developed and implanted transparent skin, through which the inner organs can be seen. It is, says one witness, 'the ultimate voyeurism.'

The machine is at the door. Is she the future?

BEYOND THE BEAUTY MYTH

Can we bring about another future, in which it is she who is dead and we who are beautifully alive?

The beauty myth countered women's new freedoms by transposing the social limits to women's lives directly onto our faces and bodies. In response, we must now ask the questions about our place in our bodies that women a generation ago asked about their place in society.

What is a woman? Is she what is made of her? Do a woman's life and experience have value? If so, should she be ashamed for them to show? What *is* so great about looking young?

The idea that a woman's body has boundaries that must not be violated is fairly new. We evidently haven't taken it far enough. Can we extend that idea? Or are women the pliable sex, innately adapted to being shaped, cut, and subjected to physical invasion? Does the female body deserve the same notion of integrity as the male body? Is there a difference between fashions in clothing and fashions in women's bodies? Assuming that someday women can be altered cheaply, painlessly, and with no risk, is that to be what we must want? Must the expressiveness of maturity and old age become extinct? Will we lose nothing if it does?

Does a woman's identity count? Must she be made to want to look like someone else? Is there something implicitly gross about the texture of female flesh? The inadequacy of female flesh stands in for the older inadequacy of the female mind. Women asserted that there was nothing inferior about their minds; are our bodies really inferior?

Is 'beauty' really sex? Does a woman's sexuality correspond to what she looks like? Does she have the right to sexual pleasure and self-esteem because she's a person, or must she earn that right through 'beauty,' as she used to through marriage? What is female sexuality – what does it look like? Does it bear any relation to the way in which commercial images represent it? Is it something women need to buy like a product? What really draws men and women together?

Are women beautiful or aren't we?

Of course we are. But we won't really believe it the way we need to until we start to take the first steps beyond the beauty myth.

Does all this mean we can't wear lipstick without feeling guilty?

On the contrary. It means we have to separate from the myth what it has surrounded and held hostage: female sexuality, bonding among women, visual enjoyment, sensual pleasure in fabrics and shapes and colors – female fun, clean and dirty. We can dissolve the myth and survive it with sex, love, attraction, and style not only intact, but flourishing more vibrantly than before. I am not attacking anything that makes women feel good; only what makes us feel bad in the first place. We all like to be desirable and feel beautiful.

But for about 160 years, middle-class, educated Western

women have been controlled by various ideals about female perfection; this old and successful tactic has worked by taking the best of female culture and attaching to it the most repressive demands of male-dominated societies. These forms of ransom were imposed on the female orgasm in the 1920s, on home and children and the family in the 1950s, on the culture of beauty in the 1980s. With this tactic, we waste time in every generation debating the symptoms more passionately than the disease.

We see this pattern of *the self-interested promotion of ideals* – eloquently pointed out in the work of Barbara Ehrenreich and Dierdre English – throughout our recent history. We must bring it up to date with the beauty myth, to get it once and for all. If we don't, as soon as we take apart the beauty myth, a new ideology will arise in its place. The beauty myth is not, ultimately, about appearance or dieting or surgery or cosmetics – any more than the Feminine Mystique was about housework. No one who is responsible for the myths of femininity in every generation really cares about the symptoms at all.

The architects of the Feminine Mystique didn't really believe that a floor in which you could see yourself indicated a cardinal virtue in women; in my own lifetime, when the idea of menstrual psychic irregularity was being clumsily resurrected as a last-ditch way to hold off the claims of the women's movement, no one was really vested in the conviction of menstrual incapacity *in itself.* By the same token, the beauty myth could not care less how much women weigh; it doesn't give a damn about the texture of women's hair or the smoothness of our skin. We intuit that, if we were all to go home tomorrow and say we never meant it really – we'll do without the jobs, the autonomy, the orgasms, the money – the beauty myth would slacken at once and grow more comfortable.

This realization makes the real issues behind the symptoms easier to see and analyze: Just as the beauty myth did not really care what women looked like as long as women felt ugly, we must see that it does not matter in the least what women look like as long as we feel beautiful.

The real issue has nothing to do with whether women wear makeup or don't, gain weight or lose it, have surgery or shun it, dress up or down, make our clothing and faces and bodies into works of art or ignore adornment altogether. *The real problem is our lack of choice.*

Under the Feminine Mystique, virtually all middle-class women were condemned to a compulsive attitude toward domesticity, whatever their individual inclinations; now that this idea is largely dismantled, those women who are personally inclined to scrupulous housekeeping pursue it, and those women who couldn't be less interested have a (relatively) greater degree of choice. We got sloppy, and the world didn't end. After we dismantle the beauty myth, a similar situation – so eminently sensible, yet so remote from where we are – will characterize our relationship to beauty culture.

The problem with cosmetics exists only when women feel invisible or inadequate without them. The problem with working out exists only if women hate ourselves when we don't. When a woman is forced to adorn herself to buy a hearing, when she needs her grooming in order to protect her identity, when she goes hungry in order to keep her job, when she must attract a lover so that she can take care of her children, that is exactly what makes 'beauty' hurt. Because what hurts women about the beauty myth is not adornment, or expressed sexuality, or time spent grooming, or the desire to attract a lover. Many mammals groom, and every culture uses adornment. 'Natural' and 'unnatural' are not the terms in question. The actual struggle is between pain and pleasure, freedom and compulsion.

Costumes and disguises will be lighthearted and fun when women are granted rock-solid identities. Clothing that highlights women's sexuality will be casual wear when women's sexuality is under our own control. When female sexuality is fully affirmed as a legitimate passion that arises from within, to be directed without stigma to the chosen object of our desire, the sexually expressive clothes or manner we may assume can no longer be used to shame us, blame us, or target us for beauty myth harassment.

The beauty myth posited to women a false choice: Which will I be, sexual or serious? We must reject that false and forced dilemma. Men's sexuality is taken to be enhanced by their seriousness; to be at the same time a serious person and a sexual being is to be fully human. Let's turn on those who offer this devil's bargain and refuse to believe that in choosing one aspect of the self we must thereby forfeit the other. In a world in which women have real choices, the choices we make about our appearance will be taken at last for what they really are: no big deal.

Women will be able thoughtlessly to adorn ourselves with pretty objects when there is no question that *we* are not objects. Women will be free of the beauty myth when we can choose to use our faces and clothes and bodies as simply one form of self-expression out of a full range of others. We can dress up for our pleasure, but we must speak up for our rights.

Many writers have tried to deal with the problems of

fantasy, pleasure, and 'glamour' by evicting them from the female Utopia. But 'glamour' is merely a demonstration of the human capacity for being enchanted, and is not in itself destructive. We need it, but redefined. We cannot disperse an exploitive religion through asceticism, or bad poetry with none at all. We can combat painful pleasure only with pure pleasure.

But let's not be naive. We are trying to make new meanings for beauty in an environment that doesn't want us to get away with it. To look however we want to look – and to be heard as we deserve to be heard – we will need no less than a feminist third wave.

Speech

The trouble with any debate about the beauty myth is the sophisticated reflex it uses: It punishes virtually any woman who tries to raise these issues by scrutinizing her appearance. It is striking to notice how thoroughly we comprehend this implied punishment. We know well how it works in a typical beauty myth double bind: No matter what a woman's appearance may be, it will be used to undermine what she is saying and taken to individualize – as her personal problem – observations she makes about aspects of the beauty myth in society.

Unfortunately, since the media routinely give accounts of women's appearance in a way that trivializes or discredits what they say, women reading or watching are routinely dissuaded from identifying with women in the public eye – the ultimate antifeminist goal of the beauty myth. Whenever we dismiss or do not hear a woman on television or in print because our attention has been drawn to her size or makeup or clothing or hairstyle, the beauty myth is working with optimum efficiency.

For a woman to go public means she must face being subjected to invasive physical scrutiny, which by definition, as we saw, no woman can pass; for a woman to speak about the beauty myth (as about women's issues in general) means that *there is no right way she can look*. There is no unmarked, or neutral, stance allowed women at those times: They are called either too 'ugly' or too 'pretty' to be believed. This reflex is working well politically: Often today, when women talk about the reasons they do not engage more with women-centered groups and movements, they often focus on differences not in agenda or worldview but in aesthetics and personal style. By keeping the antifeminist origins and reactionary purpose of this direction of attention always in mind, we can thwart the myth. For us to reject the insistence that a woman's appearance *is her speech,* for us to hear one another out beyond the beauty myth, is itself a political step forward.

Blame

Blame is what fuels the beauty myth; to take it apart, let us refuse forever to blame ourselves and other women for what it, in its great strength, has tried to do. The most important change to aim at is this: When someone tries, in the future, to use the beauty myth against us, we will no longer look in the mirror to see what we have done wrong. Women can organize around discrimination in employment on the basis of appearance only when we examine the usual reactions to such complaints ('Well, why did you wear that tight sweater?' 'So, why don't you do something about yourself?') and reject them. We cannot speak up about the myth until we believe in our guts that there is nothing objective about how the myth works – that when women are called too ugly or too pretty to do something we want to do, this has nothing to do with our appearance. Women can summon the courage to talk about the myth in public by keeping in mind that attacks on or flattery of our appearance in public are never at fault. It is all impersonal; it is political.

The reflexive responses that have developed to keep us silent will doubtless increase in intensity: 'Easy for you to say.' 'You're too pretty to be a feminist.' 'No wonder she's a feminist; look at her.' 'What does she expect, dressed like that?'

'That's what comes of vanity.' 'What makes you think they were whistling at you?' 'What was she wearing?' 'Don't you wish.' 'Don't flatter yourself.' 'There's no excuse any more for a woman to look her age.' 'Sour grapes?' 'A bimbo.' 'Brainless.' 'She's using it for all she can get.' Recognizing these reactions for what they are, it may be easier to brave coercive flattery or insults or both, and make some long-overdue scenes.

This will be hard. Talking about the beauty myth strikes a nerve which, for most of us, is on some level very raw. We will need to have compassion for ourselves and other women for our strong feelings about 'beauty,' and be very gentle with those feelings. If the beauty myth is religion, it is because women still lack rituals that include us; if it is economy, it is because we're still compensated unfairly; if it is sexuality, it is because female sexuality is still a dark continent; if it is warfare, it is because women are denied ways to see ourselves as heroines, daredevils, stoics, and rebels;

if it is women's culture, it is because men's culture still resists us. When we recognize that the myth is powerful because it has claimed so much of the best of female consciousness, we can turn from it to look more clearly at all it has tried to stand in for.

A Feminist Third Wave

So here we are. What can we do?

We must dismantle the PBQ; support the unionization of women's jobs; make 'beauty' harassment, age discrimination, unsafe working conditions such as enforced surgery, and the double standard for appearance, issues for labor negotiation; women in television and other heavily discriminatory professions must organize for wave after wave of lawsuits; we must insist on equal enforcement of dress codes, take a deep breath, and tell our stories.

It is often said that we must make fashion and advertising images include us, but this is a dangerously optimistic misunderstanding of how the market works. Advertising aimed at women works by lowering our self-esteem. If it flatters our self-esteem, it is not effective. Let's abandon this hope of looking to the index fully to include us. It won't, because if it does, it has lost its function. As long as the definition of 'beauty' comes from outside women, we will continue to be manipulated by it.

We claimed the freedom to age and remain sexual, but that rigidified into the condition of aging 'youthfully.' We began to wear comfortable clothing, but the discomfort settled back onto our bodies. The seventies' 'natural' beauty became its own icon; the 1980s' 'healthy' beauty brought about an epidemic of new diseases and 'strength as beauty' enslaved women to our muscles. This process will continue with every effort women make to reform the index until we change our relationship to the index altogether.

The marketplace is not open to consciousness-raising. It is misplaced energy to attack the market's images themselves: Given recent history, they were bound to develop as they did.

While we cannot directly affect the images, we can drain them of their power. We can turn away from them, look directly at one another, and find alternative images of beauty in a female subculture; seek out the plays, music, films that illuminate women in three dimensions; find the biographies of women, the women's history, the heroines that in each generation are submerged from view; fill in the terrible, 'beautiful' blanks. We can lift ourselves and other women out of the myth – but only if we are willing to seek out and support and really look at the alternatives.

Since our imaginary landscape fades to gray when we try to think past the myth, women need cultural help to imagine our way free. For most of our history, the representation of women, our sexuality and our true beauty, has not been in our hands. After just twenty years of the great push foward, during which time women sought to define those things for ourselves, the marketplace, more influential than any solitary artist, has seized the definition of our desire. Shall we let women-hating images claim our sexuality for their royalties? We need to insist on making culture out of our desire: making paintings, novels, plays, and films potent and seductive and authentic enough to undermine and overwhelm the Iron Maiden. Let's expand our culture to separate sex from the Iron Maiden.

We'll need to remember, at the same time, how heavily

censored our mass culture is by beauty advertisers: As long as primetime TV and the mainstream press aimed at women are supported by beauty advertisers, the story line of how women are in mass culture will be dictated by the beauty myth. It is understood without directives that stories that center admiringly on an 'unprocessed' woman will rarely get made. If we could see a sixty-year-old woman who looks her age read the news, a deep fissure would open in the beauty myth. Meanwhile, let's be clear that the myth rules the airwaves *only* because the products of the process buy the time.

Finally, we can keep our analytical gaze always sharp, being aware of what shapes the Iron Maiden can affect how we see, absorb, and respond to her images. Quickly, with this consciousness, they begin to look like what they are – two-dimensional. They literally fall flat. It is when they become tedious to us that they will evolve to *adapt* to the sea change in women's moods; an advertiser can't influence a story line if there is no audience. Responding to sheer boredom on women's part, creators of culture will be forced to present three-dimensional images of women in order to involve us again. Women can provoke, through our sudden boredom with the Iron Maiden, a mass culture that does in fact treat us like people.

In transforming the cultural environment, women who work in the mainstream media are a crucial inside vanguard. I have heard many women in the media express frustration at the limitations surrounding the treatment of beauty myth issues; many report a sense of isolation in relation to pushing those limits. Perhaps debate renewed in more political terms about the beauty myth in the media, and the seriousness of its consequences, will forge new alliances in support of those women in print and TV and radio journalism who are eager to battle the beauty myth at ground zero.

Quickly, when we put together a personal counterculture of meaningful images of beauty, the Iron Maiden begins to look like an image of unattractive violence; alternative ways to see start to leap out from the background.

The beauty cult attests to a spiritual hunger for female ritual and rites of passage. We need to develop and elaborate better women's rituals to fill in the void. Can we evolve more widely among friends, among networks of friends, fruitful new rites and celebrations for the female life cycle? We have baby showers and bridal showers, but what about purification, confirmation, healing, and renewal ceremonies for childbirth, first menstruation, loss of virginity, graduation, first job, marriage, recovery from heartbreak or divorce, the earning of a degree, menopause? Whatever organic form they take, we need new and positive, rather than negative, celebrations to mark the female lifespan.

To protect our sexuality from the beauty myth, we can believe in the importance of cherishing, nurturing, and attending to our sexuality as to an animal or a child. Sexuality is not inert or given but, like a living being, changes with what it feeds upon. We can stay away from gratuitously sexually violent or exploitive images – and, when we do encounter them, ask ourselves to feel them as such. We can seek out those dreams and visions that include a sexuality free of exploitation or violence, and try to stay as conscious of what we take into our imaginations as we now are of what enters our bodies.

An eroticism of equality may be hard to visualize now. Critiques of sexuality tend to stop short with the assumption that sexuality cannot evolve. But for most women, fantasies of objectification or violence are learned superficially through a patina of images. I believe that they can be as easily unlearned by consciously reversing our conditioning – by making the repeated association between pleasure and mutuality. Our ideas of sexual beauty are open to more transformation than we yet realize.

We need, especially for the anorexic/pornographic generations, a radical rapprochement with nakedness. Many women have described the sweeping revelation that follows even one experience of communal all-female nakedness. This is an easy suggestion to mock, but the fastest way to demystify the naked Iron Maiden is to promote retreats, festivals, excursions, that include – whether in swimming or sunning or Turkish baths or random relaxation – communal nakedness. Men's groups, from fraternities to athletic clubs, understand the value, the cohesiveness, and the esteem for one's own gender generated by such moments. A single revelation of the beauty of our infinite variousness is worth more than words; one such experience is strong enough, for a young girl, especially, to give the lie to the Iron Maiden.

When faced with the myth, the questions to ask are not about women's faces and bodies but about the power relations of the situation. Who is this serving? Who says? Who profits? What is the context? When someone discusses a woman's appearance to her face, she can ask herself, Is it that person's business? Are the power relations equal? Would she feel comfortable making the same personal comments in return?

A woman's appearance is more often called to her attention for a political reason than as a constituent of genuine attraction and desire. We can learn to get better at telling the difference – a liberating skill in itself. We need not condemn lust, seduction, or physical attraction – a much more democratic and subjective quality than the market would like us to discover – we need only to reject political manipulation.

The irony is that more beauty promises what only more female solidarity can deliver: The beauty myth can be defeated for good only through an electric resurgence of the woman-centered political activism of the seventies – a feminist third wave – updated to take on the new issues of the nineties. In this decade, for young women in particular, some of the enemies are quieter and cleverer and harder to grasp. To enlist young women, we'll need to define our self-esteem as political: to rank it, along with money, jobs, child care, safety, as a vital resource for women that is *deliberately* kept in inadequate supply.

I don't pretend to have the agenda; I know only that some of the problems have changed. I've become convinced that there are thousands of young women ready and eager to join forces with a peer-driven feminist third wave that would take on, along with the classic feminist agenda, the new problems that have arisen with the shift in *Zeitgeist* and the beauty backlash. The movement would need to deal with the ambiguities of assimilation. Young women express feelings of being scared and isolated 'insiders' as opposed to angry and united outsiders, and this distinction makes backlash sense: The best way to stop a revolution is to give people something to lose. It would need to politicize eating disorders, young women's uniquley intense relationship to images, and the effect of those images on their sexuality – it would need to make the point that you don't have much of a right over your own body if you can't eat. It would need to analyze the antifeminist propaganda young women have inherited, and give them tools, including arguments like this one, with which to see through it. While transmitting the previous heritage of feminism intact, it would need to be, as all feminist waves are, peer-driven: No matter how wise a mother's advice is, we listen to our peers. It would have to make joy, rowdiness, and wanton celebration as much a part of its project as hard work and bitter struggle, and it can begin all this by rejecting the pernicious fib that is crippling young women – the fib called postfeminism, the pious hope that the battles have all been won. This scary word is making young women, who face many of the same old problems, once again blame themselves – since it's all been fixed, right? It strips them of the weapon of theory and makes them feel alone once again. We never speak complacently of the post-Democratic era: Democracy, we know, is a living, vulnerable thing that every generation must renew. The same goes for that aspect of democracy represented by feminism. So let's get on with it.

Women learned to crave 'beauty' in its contemporary form because we were learning at the same time that the feminist struggle was going to be much harder than we had realized. The ideology of 'beauty' was a shortcut promise to agitating women – a historical placebo – that we could be confident, valued, heard out, respected, and make demands without fear. (In fact, it is doubtful whether 'beauty' is the real desire at all; women may want 'beauty' so that we can get back inside their bodies, and crave perfection so that we can forget about the whole damn thing. Most women, in their guts, would probably rather be, given the choice, a sexual, courageous self than a beautiful generic Other.)

Beauty advertising copy promises that sort of courage

and freedom – 'Beachwear for the beautiful and brave'; 'A fresh, fearless look,' 'A funky fearlessness'; 'Think radical'; 'The Freedom Fighters – for the woman who isn't afraid to speak up or stand out.' But this courage and confidence will not be real until we are backed by the material gains that we can achieve only by seeing other women as allies rather than as competitors.

The 1980s tried to buy us off with promises of individual solutions. We have reached the limit of what the individualist, beauty-myth version of female progress can do, and it is not good enough: We will be 2 percent of top management and 5 percent of full professors and 5 percent of senior partners forever if we do not get together for the next great push forward. Higher cheekbones and firmer bustlines clearly won't get us what we need for real confidence and visibility; only a renewed commitment to the basics of female political progress – to childcare programs, effective antidiscrimination laws, parental leave, reproductive choice, fair compensation, and genuine penalties against sexual violence – will do so. We won't have these until we can identify our interests in other women's, and allow our natural solidarity to overcome the organizational obstacles put forward by the competitiveness and rivalry artificially provoked among us by the beauty backlash.

The terrible truth is that though the marketplace promotes the myth, it would be powerless if women didn't enforce it against one another. For any one woman to outgrow the myth, she needs the support of many women. The toughest but most necessary change will come not from men or from the media, but from women, in the way we see and behave toward other women.

Generational Collaboration

The links between generations of women need mending if we are to save one another from the beauty myth, and save women's progress from its past historical fate – the periodic reinvention of the wheel. Gill Hudson, editor of *Company*, reveals the extent to which the beauty backlash has propagandized the young: Young women, she says, 'absolutely don't want to be known as feminists' because 'feminism is not considered sexy.' It would be stupid and sad if the women of the near future had to fight the same old battles all over again from the beginning just because of young women's isolation from older women. It would be pathetic if young women had to go back to the beginning because we were taken in by an unoriginal twenty-year campaign to portray the women's movement as 'not sexy,' a campaign aimed to help young women forget whose battles made sex sexy in the first place.

Since young women will not be encouraged by our institutions to make the connections, we can get past the myth only by actively exploring more useful role models than the glossies give us. We are sorely in need of intergenerational contact: We need to see the faces of the women who made our freedom possible; they need to hear our thanks. Young women are dangerously 'unmothered' – unprotected, unguided – institutionally and need role models and mentors. The work and experience of older women gain scope and influence when imparted to students, apprentices, protégés. Yet, both generations will have to resist their externally ingrained impulses against intergenerational collaboration. We are well trained, if young, to shy away from identification with older women; if older, at being a little hard on young women, viewing them with impatience and disdain. The beauty myth is designed artifically to pit the generations of women against one another; our consciously strengthening those links gives back the wholeness of our lifespans that the beauty myth would keep us from discovering.

Divide and Conquer

The fact is, women are not actually dangerous to one another. Outside the myth, other women look a lot like natural allies. In order for women to learn to fear one another, we had to be convinced that our sisters possess some kind of mysterious, potent secret weapon to be used against us – the imaginary weapon being 'beauty.'

The core of the myth – and the reason it was so useful as a counter to feminism – is its divisiveness. You can see and hear it everywhere: 'Don't hate me because I'm beautiful' (L'Oréal). 'I really hate my aerobics instructor – I guess hatred is good motivation.' 'You'd hate her. She has everything.' 'Women who get out of bed looking beautiful really annoy me.' 'Don't you hate women who can eat like that?' 'No pores – makes you sick.' 'Tall, blonde – couldn't you just kill her?' Rivalry, resentment, and hostility provoked by the beauty myth run deep. Sisters commonly remember the grief of one being designated 'the pretty one.' Mothers often have difficulty with their daughters' blooming. Jealousy among the best of friends is a cruel fact of female love. Even women who are lovers describe beauty competition. It is painful for women to talk about beauty because under the myth, one woman's body is used to hurt another. Our faces and bodies become instruments for punishing other women, often used out of our control and against our will. At present, 'beauty' is an economy in which women find the 'value' of their faces and bodies impinging, in spite of themselves, on that of other women's. This constant comparison, in which one woman's worth fluctuates through the presence of another, divides and conquers. It forces women to be acutely critical of the 'choices' other women make about how they look. But that economy that pits women against one another is not inevitable.

To get past this divisiveness, women will have to break a lot of taboos against talking about it, including the one that prohibits women from narrating the dark side of being treated as a beautiful object. From the dozens of women to whom I have listened, it is clear that the amount of pain a given woman experiences through the beauty myth bears no relationship at all to what she looks like relative to a cultural ideal. (In the words of a top fashion model, 'When I was on the cover of the Italian *Vogue,* everyone told me how great I looked. I just thought, "I can't believe you can't see all those lines."') Women who impersonate the Iron Maiden may be no less victimized by the myth than the women subjected to their images. The myth asks women to be at once blindly hostile to and blindly envious of 'beauty' in other women. Both the hostility and the envy serve the myth and hurt all women.

While the 'beautiful' woman is briefly at the apex of the system, this is, of course, far from the divine state of grace that the myth propagates. The pleasure to be had from turning oneself into a living art object, the roaring in the ears and the fine jetspray of regard on the surface of the skin, is some kind of power, when power is in short supply. But it is not much compared to the pleasure of getting back forever inside the body; the pleasure of discovering sexual pride, a delight in a common female sexuality that overwhelms the divisions of 'beauty'; the pleasure of shedding self-consciousness and narcissism and guilt like a chainmail gown; the pleasure of the freedom to forget all about it.

Only then will women be able to talk about what 'beauty' really involves: the attention of people we do not know, rewards for things we did not earn, sex from men who reach for us as for a brass ring on a carousel, hostility and scepticism from other women, adolescence extended longer than it ought to be, cruel aging, and a long hard struggle for identity. And we will learn that what is good about 'beauty' – the promise of confidence, sexuality, and the self-regard of a healthy individuality – are actually qualities that have nothing to do with 'beauty' specifically, but are deserved by and, as the myth is dismantled, available to all women. The best that 'beauty' offers belongs to us all by right of femaleness. When we separate 'beauty' from sexuality, when we celebrate the individuality of our features and characteristics, women will have access to a pleasure in our bodies that unites us rather than divides us. The beauty myth will be history.

But as long as women censor in one another the truths about our experiences, 'beauty' will remain mystified and still most useful to those who wish to control women. The unacceptable reality is that we live under a caste system. It is not innate and permanent; it is not based on sex or God or the Rock of Ages. It can and must be changed. The situation is closing in on us, and there is no long term left to which to postpone the conversation.

When the conversation commences, the artificial barriers of the myth will begin to fall away. We will hear that just because a woman looks 'beautiful' doesn't mean she feels it, and she can feel beautiful without looking it at first glance. Thin women may feel fat; young women will grow old.

When one woman looks at another, she cannot possibly know the self-image within that woman: Though she appears enviably in control, she may be starving; though she overflows her clothing, she may be enviably satisfied sexually. A woman may be fleshy from high self-esteem or from low; she may cover her face in makeup out of the desire to play around outrageously or the desire to hide. All women have experienced the world treating them better or worse according to where they rate each day: while this experience wreaks havoc with a woman's identity, it does mean that women have access to a far greater range of experience than the snapshots 'beauty' takes of us would lead us to believe. We may well discover that the way we now read appearances tells us little, and that we experience, no matter what we look like, the same spectrum of feelings: sometimes lovely, often unlovely, always female, in a commonality that extends across the infinite grids that the beauty myth tries to draw among us.

Women blame men for looking but not listening. But we do it too; perhaps even more so. We have to stop reading each others' appearances as if appearance were language, political allegiance, worthiness, or aggression. The chances are excellent that what a woman means to say *to other women* is far more complex and sympathetic than the garbled message that her appearance permits her.

Let us start with a reinterpretation of 'beauty' that is *noncompetitive, nonhierarchical, and nonviolent.* Why must one woman's pleasure and pride have to mean another woman's pain? Men are only in sexual competition when they are competing sexually, but the myth puts women in 'sexual' competition in every situation. Competition for a specific sexual partner is rare; since it is not usually a competition 'for men,' it is not biologically inevitable.

Women compete this way 'for other women' partly because we are devotees of the same sect, and partly to fill, if only temporarily, the black hole that the myth created in the first place. Hostile competition can often be proof of what our current sexual arrangements repress: our mutual physical attraction. If women redefine sexuality to affirm our attraction among ourselves, the myth will no longer hurt. Other women's beauty will not be a threat or an insult, but a pleasure and a tribute. Women will be able to costume and adorn ourselves without fear of hurting and betraying other women, or of being accused of false loyalties. We can then dress up in celebration of the shared pleasure of the female body, doing it 'for other women' in a positive rather than a negative offering of the self.

And when we let ourselves experience this physical attraction, the marketplace will no longer be able to make a profit out of its representation of men's desires: We, knowing firsthand that attraction to other women comes in many forms, will no longer believe that the qualities that make us desirable are a lucrative mystery.

By changing our prejudgments of one another, we have the means for the beginning of a noncompetitive experience of beauty. The 'other woman' is represented through the myth as an unknown danger. 'Meet the Other Woman,' reads a Wella hair-coloring brochure, referring to the 'after' version of the woman targeted. The idea is that 'beauty' makes *another* woman – even one's own idealized image – into a being so alien that you need a formal introduction. It is a phrase that suggests threats, mistresses, glamorous destroyers of relationships.

We undo the myth by approaching the unknown Other

Woman. Since women's everyday experiences of flirtatious attention derive most often from men reacting to our 'beauty,' it is no wonder that silent, watching women can be represented to us as antagonists.

We can melt this suspicion and distance: Why should we not be gallant and chivalrous and flirtatious with one another. Let us charm one another with some of that sparkling attention too often held in reserve only for men: compliment one another, show our admiration. We can engage with the Other Woman – catch her eye, give her a lift when she is hitchhiking, open the door when she is struggling. When we approach one another in the street and give, or receive, that wary, defensive shoes-to-haircut glance, what if we meet one another's eyes woman to woman; what if we smile.

This movement toward a noncompetitive idea of beauty is already underway. The myth has always denied women honor. Here and there, women are evolving codes of honor to protect us from it. We withold easy criticism. We shower authentic praise. We bow out of social situations in which our beauty is being used to put other women in the shadows. We refuse to jostle for random male attention. A contestant in the 1989 Miss California Pageant pulls a banner from her swimsuit that reads PAGEANTS HURT ALL WOMEN. A film actress tells me that when she did a nude scene, she refused, as a gesture to women in the audience, to discipline her body first. We are already beginning to find ways in which we won't be rivals and we won't be instruments.

This new perspective changes not how we look but how we see. We begin to see other women's faces and bodies for themselves, the Iron Maiden no longer superimposed. We catch our breath when we see a woman laughing. We cheer inside when we see a woman walk proud. We smile in the mirror, watch the lines form at the corners of our eyes, and, pleased with what we are making, smile again.

Though women can give this new perspective to one another, men's participation in overturning the myth is welcome. Some men, certainly, have used the beauty myth abusively against women, the way some men use their fists; but there is a strong consciousness among both sexes that the real agents enforcing the myth today are not men as individual lovers or husbands, but institutions, that depend on male dominance. Both sexes seem to be finding that the full force of the myth derives little from private sexual relations, and much from the cultural and economic megalith 'out there' in the public realm. Increasingly, both sexes know they are being cheated.

But helping women to take the myth apart is in men's own interest on an even deeper level: Their turn is next. Advertisers have recently figured out that undermining sexual self-confidence works whatever the targeted gender. According to *The Guardian,* 'Men are now looking at mirrors instead of at girls...Beautiful men can now be seen selling everything.' Using images from male homosexual subculture, advertising has begun to portray the male body in a beauty myth of its own. As this imagery focuses more closely on male sexuality, it will undermine the sexual self-esteem of men in general. Since men are more conditioned to be separate from their bodies, and to compete to inhuman excess, the male version could conceivably hurt men even more than the female version hurts women.

Psychiatrists are anticipating a rise in male rates of eating diseases. Now that men are being cast as a frontier market to be opened up by self-hatred, images have begun to tell heterosexual men the same halftruths about what women want and how they see that they have traditionally told heterosexual women about men; if they buy it and become trapped themselves, that will be no victory for women. No one will win.

But it is also in men's interest to undo the myth because the survival of the planet depends on it. The earth can no longer afford a consumer ideology based on the insatiable wastefulness of sexual and material discontent. We need to begin to get lasting satisfaction out of the things we consume. We conceived of the planet as female, an all-giving Mother Nature, just as we conceived of the female body, infinitely alterable by and for man; we serve both ourselves and our hopes for the planet by insisting on a new female reality on which to base a new metaphor for the earth: the female body with its own organic integrity that must be respected.

The environmental crisis demands a new way of thinking that is communitarian, collective and not adversarial, and we need it fast. We can pray and hope that male institutions evolve this sophisticated, unfamiliar way of thinking within a few short years; or we can turn to the female tradition, which has perfected it over five millennia, and adapt it to the public sphere. Since the beauty myth blots out the female tradition, we keep a crucial option for the planet open when we resist it.

And we keep options open for ourselves. We do not need to change our bodies, we need to change the rules. Beyond the myth, women will still be blamed for our appearances by whom ever needs to blame us. So let's stop blaming ourselves and stop running and stop apologizing, and let's start to please ourselves once and for all. The 'beautiful' woman does not win under the myth; neither does anyone else. The woman who is subjected to the continual adulation of strangers does not win, nor does the woman who denies herself attention. The woman who wears a uniform does not win, nor does the woman with a designer outfit for every day of the year. You do not win by struggling to the top of a caste system, you win by refusing to be trapped within one at all. The woman wins who calls herself beautiful and challenges the world to change to truly see her.

A woman wins by giving herself and other women permission – to eat; to be sexual; to age; to wear overalls, a paste tiara, a Balenciaga gown, a second-hand opera cloak, or combat boots; to cover up or to go practically naked; to do whatever we choose in following – or ignoring – our own aesthetic. A woman wins when she feels that what each woman does with her own body – unforced, uncoerced – is her own business. When many individual women exempt themselves from the economy, it will begin to dissolve. Institutions, some men, and some women, will continue to try to use women's appearance against us. But we won't bite.

Can there be a pro-woman definition of beauty? Absolutely. What has been missing is play. The beauty myth is harmful and pompous and grave because so much, too much, depends upon it. The pleasure of playfulness is that it doesn't matter. Once you play for stakes of any amount, the game becomes a war game, or compulsive gambling. In the myth, it has been a game for life, for questionable love, for desperate and dishonest sexuality, and without the choice not to play by alien rules. No choice, no free will; no levity, no real game.

But we can imagine, to save ourselves, a life in the body that is not value-laden; a masquerade, a voluntary theatricality that emerges from abundant self-love. A pro-woman redefinition of beauty reflects our redefinitions of what power is. Who says we need a hierarchy? Where I see beauty may not be where you do. Some people look more desirable to me than they do to you. So what? My perception has no authority over yours. Why should beauty be exclusive? Admiration can include so much. Why is rareness impressive? The high value of rareness is a masculine concept, having more to do with capitalism than with lust. What is the fun in wanting the most what cannot be found? Children, in contrast, are common as dirt, but they are highly valued and regarded as beautiful.

How might women act beyond the myth? Who can say? Maybe we will let our bodies wax and wane, enjoying the variations on a theme, and avoid pain because when something hurts us it begins to look ugly to us. Maybe we will adorn ourselves with real delight, with the sense that we are gilding the lily. Maybe the less pain women inflict on our bodies, the more beautiful our bodies will look to us. Perhaps we will forget to elicit admiration from strangers, and find we don't miss it; perhaps we will await our older faces with anticipation, and be unable to see our bodies as a mass of imperfections, since there is nothing on us that is not precious. Maybe we won't want to be the 'after' anymore.

How to begin? Let's be shameless. Be greedy. Pursue pleasure. Avoid pain. Wear and touch and eat and drink what we feel like. Tolerate other women's choices. Seek out the sex we want and fight fiercely against the sex we do not want. Choose our own causes. And once we break through and change the rules so our sense of our own beauty cannot be shaken, sing that beauty and dress it up and flaunt it and revel in it: In a sensual politics, female is beautiful.

A woman-loving definition of beauty supplants desperation with play, narcissism with self-love, dismemberment with wholeness, absence with presence, stillness with animation. It admits radiance: light coming out of the face and the body, rather than a spotlight on the body, dimming the self. It is sexual, various, and surprising. We will be able to see it in others and not be frightened, and able at last to see it in ourselves.

A generation ago, Germaine Greer wondered about women: 'What *will* you do?' What women did brought about a quarter century of cataclysmic social revolution. The next phase of our movement forward as individual women, as women together, and as tenants of our bodies and this planet, depends now on what we decide to see when we look in the mirror.

What *will* we see?

ACKNOWLEDGMENTS

I owe this book to the support of my family: Leonard and Deborah and Aaron Wolfe, Daniel Goleman, Tara Bennet-Goleman, Anasuya Weil and Tom Weil. I'm expecially grateful to my grandmother, Fay Goleman, on whose unflagging encouragement I depended and whose life – as family services pioneer, professor, wife, mother, and early feminist – gives continual inspiration. I'm grateful to Ruth Sullivan, Esther Boner, Lily Rivlin, Michele Landsberg, Joanne Stewart, Florence Lewis, Patricia Pierce, Alan Shoaf, Polly Shulman, Elizabeth Alexander, Rhonda Garelick, Amruta Slee, and Barbara Browning for their vital contributions to my work. Jane Meara and Jim Landis gave their thoughtful editorial attention very generously. Colin Troup was a ready source of comfort, contentiousness, and amusement. And I am indebted to the theorists of femininity of the second wave, without whose struggles with these issues I could not have begun my own.

THE HISTORY OF VINTAGE

The famous American publisher Alfred A. Knopf (1892–1984) founded Vintage Books in the United States in 1954 as a paperback home for the authors published by his company. Vintage was launched in the United Kingdom in 1990 and works independently from the American imprint although both are part of the international publishing group, Random House.

Vintage in the United Kingdom was initially created to publish paperback editions of books bought by the prestigious literary hardback imprints in the Random House Group such as Jonathan Cape, Chatto & Windus, Hutchinson and later William Heinemann, Secker & Warburg and The Harvill Press. There are many Booker and Nobel Prize-winning authors on the Vintage list and the imprint publishes a huge variety of fiction and non-fiction. Over the years Vintage has expanded and the list now includes great authors of the past – who are published under the Vintage Classics imprint – as well as many of the most influential authors of the present. In 2012 Vintage Children's Classics was launched to include the much-loved authors of our youth.

For a full list of the books Vintage publishes,
please visit our website
www.vintage-books.co.uk

For book details and other information about the classic authors we publish, please visit the Vintage Classics website
www.vintage-classics.info

www.vintage-classics.info

Visit www.worldofstories.co.uk for all your
favourite children's classics